Vertical Athlete

Fundamentals of Training for Pole Fitness and Dance

Bethany Freel

Vertical Athlete: Fundamentals of Training for Pole Fitness and Dance by Bethany Freel

Published by: Poler North, Anchorage, Alaska

Library of Congress Control Number: 2013905649

ISBN-13: 978-0615791470
ISBN-10: 0615791476

For discounts on bulk orders and for additional information please contact the publisher at info@polernorth.com or visit www.verticalathletepoletraining.com

"You are unrepeatable. There is a magic about you that is all your own."

–D. M. Dellinger

To all of you unique and remarkable polers out there!

Contents

Introduction

The ultimate goal of any training program is to induce physiological and psychological alterations resulting in increased athletic performance. In other words, people train to get better at what they are doing. Even those who train simply for the health benefits expect to see progress in their performance. Today we are surrounded by a myriad of exercise and training prescriptions through books, magazines, well-meaning friends, celebrities, and the media in general. Unfortunately, much of this information is more based on fad than fact. Because each person and each sport are unique, fad exercise programs can be dangerous and unproductive means to train. In order for an athlete to avoid overtraining and reach their true performance potential, they must train with a knowledge and awareness of their own body, their sport, and the fundamental principles of training.

To the benefit of many, pole fitness and dance is quickly growing around the world. Thousands of budding athletes have gained impressive strength and skill. Women and men from countless backgrounds are experiencing an enjoyable, expressive form of exercise. As the numerous positive aspects of pole become more apparent to the world and elite performance grows more advanced, it is especially important for current and aspiring athletes to be knowledgeable in the best ways to train for pole. The following chapters provide the essential components of a successful pole training program. With awareness and application of cultural influences, physiology, principles of training, overtraining, and program design, a person at any current training level can reach amazing levels of athletic performance.

Chapter 1
Cultural Influences on Training

Fitness and performance enhancements in sport come from a combination of applied training stress and rest. Unfortunately, the later and perhaps more important component, rest, is rarely emphasized or even mentioned in our society. Perhaps this is because rest isn't something we actively do. Our society is very task oriented, focused on accomplishing things in the most productive and efficient way.   A headline article in a pop culture exercise magazine suggesting snuggling on the couch for a television marathon after a week of training would seem repulsive to the "get better by doing more" attitude. The physical exercise portion of training is the part where we <u>do</u> something, so when we see positive results, it's easy to assume that these are due to the training stresses we applied to our bodies. Rest or any non-exercise activity is then seen as unproductive in terms of performance enhance-

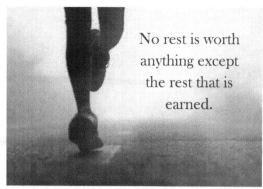

No rest is worth anything except the rest that is earned.

ment. Instead of emphasizing the importance of both components of training, we are bombarded by problematic, misconstrued messages that more exercise is always better, that we have to be in pain to experience gains in performance, that rest is for the weak. To the athlete unaware of proper training theory and methodology, these messages can result in a training program that causes frequent injury, fatigue, emotional trauma, and performance stagnation or loss.

When it comes to weight, size, and superficial image, our society's value system doesn't help the situation either. Huge significance is often placed on how a person looks and performs either directly by coaches, fans, demanding parents, etc., or indirectly through the media, popular figures, and other individuals. With such emphasis on image, individuals often associate their personal worth or value based on how they look. In a desire to be loved and accepted, a person may go to whatever extremes necessary to attain the idealized "fit" appearance that has become idolized in our society. An IDEA fitness publication from 2005, for example,

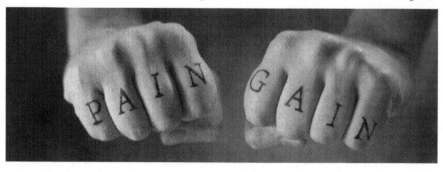

reported that 19% of overweight people would risk death to be thin and 33% of obese people would do the same to lose just 10 pounds (2)!

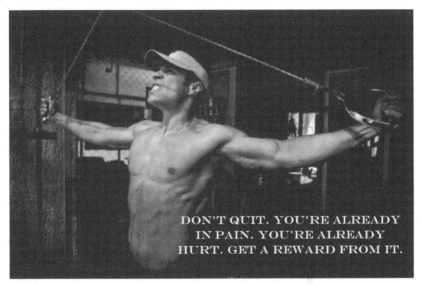

DON'T QUIT. YOU'RE ALREADY IN PAIN. YOU'RE ALREADY HURT. GET A REWARD FROM IT.

It's no wonder that these levels of desperation to reach perfection could lead to damaging levels of overtraining in athletes. In addition to such emphasis on image, athletes are also faced with a culture that treats pain and injury as a badge of honor. Injury is often seen as a measure of an athlete's dedication and training effort. It is rare to see an athlete esteemed for a symptom free season due to an extra dose of rest and recovery. Instead, we label a hero the one who limped to the end of the race with a stress fracture in their leg. To the unaware or particularly driven athlete, this emphasizes cultural imperatives like "no-pain, no-gain" and grossly and dangerously perpetuates the distortion of a stress/recovery balance in athletic training.

Over the years, harmful societal influences have become deeply rooted in many athletic activities (4, 5). Fortunately, most pole athletes are obviously not held back by the idea of traditional social acceptance. With attitudes that circumvent what is considered acceptable and what is not, there is an amazing opportunity in the pole community to create and sustain an environment that dismisses inaccurate and harmful ideas about training, body image, and self-worth and instead fosters constructive athletic training practices and personal growth. Not only will this promote emotional health and well-being, it will also result in superior athletic performance. With an accurate base of knowledge in how the body works and the fundamentals of athletic training, many of the destructive popular training practices can be avoided, allowing each individual athlete to rise to their true potential.

Continuing Education Questions

1. What are some of the possible negative outcomes of today's popular training imperatives?
2. What component of an athletic training program is emphasized most in today's society?
3. List some of the popular sayings/imperatives that influence current perspectives on training and exercise.
4. What are some of the possible opportunities in the growing pole community with respect to training theory and methodology and socially driven perceptions?

References and Additional Sources

1. Beard, A., & Paley, R. (2012). In the water they can't see you cry: A memoir. New York, NY: Simon & Schuster.
2. Lofshult, D. (2005). Dying to be thin. IDEA Fitness Journal, 2 (5).
3. Meyers, A. W., & Whelan, J. P. (1998). A systemic model for understanding psychosocial influences in overtraining. In R. B. Kreider, A. C. Fry, & M. L. O'Toole (Eds.), Overtraining in sport (pp. 335-364). Champaign, IL: Human Kinetics.

4. Richardson, S. O., Andersen, M. B., & Morris, T. (2008). Overtraining athletes: Personal journeys in sport. Champaign, IL: Human Kinetics.
5. Stamford, B. A., & Shimer, P. (1990). Fitness without exercise: The scientifically proven strategy for achieving maximum health with minimum effort. New York, NY: Warner Books.

Chapter 2

Sports Physiology

Muscles and the Nervous System

There are three main different types of muscles in the body. One is smooth muscle. This is the type of muscle that makes up the stomach, intestines, and blood vessels. These are typically controlled involuntarily and help to regulate movement of fluid and materials throughout the body. A second type, cardiac muscle, forms the wall of the heart. It is also involuntarily controlled by the body but has an alternating light/dark striated appearance not found in smooth muscle. The third type, skeletal muscle, is often the type of muscle referred to when talking about muscle in the context of athletics and exercise.

Skeletal muscles are like Russian Matryoshka nesting dolls. When we examine the outside of a muscle we are looking at an

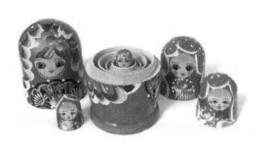

external tissue casing called fascia. The outermost fascia is called the epimysium. The epimysium, like the largest Matryoshka doll, incases smaller muscle bundles wrapped up in another layer of fascia called the Perimysium. Inside the Perimysium we find small bundles of muscle fibers called fasciculi. This nested structure of thousands of muscle fibers allows even small muscles to create immense forces. But how do these fibers create force? To answer that question we have to go even deeper within the muscle Matryoshka.

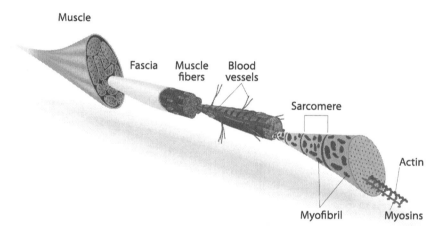

Each muscle fiber itself contains hundreds of threadlike protein strands called myofibrils which in turn contain thousands of microscopic myofilaments. It is these tiny, nearly invisible protein filaments that cumulatively create the force to both push the snooze button and perform a twisted grip dead lift. There are two different myofilaments that create muscular force. These tiny strands called Actin and Myosin alternate within the myofibril, overlapping at their edges. Each repeated section of Actin and Myosin is collectively called a Sarcomere. Attached to the Myosin are tiny protein projections called cross-bridges. These reach out towards the Actin filaments and when sufficient energy is present in the muscle, their free ends attach and pull the Actin filaments in toward the center of the Myosin. As each Actin filament is pulled inward toward the center of the Myosin filaments, the myofibril scrunches. Since each skeletal muscle is ultimately made of bundles of myofilaments, this scrunching results in muscle scrunching, better known as muscle contraction. All the names and big words aside, a skeletal muscle is just a bundle of bundles of even smaller bundles of fibers which all scrunch together to create contraction.

Skeletal muscles are attached to bones, but not directly. At each end of a typical skeletal muscle is a tendon which is in turn connected to bone. Tendons are made of a much stronger, less elastic material called collagen. This enables them to transmit great force to the skeletal system but also makes them more susceptible to

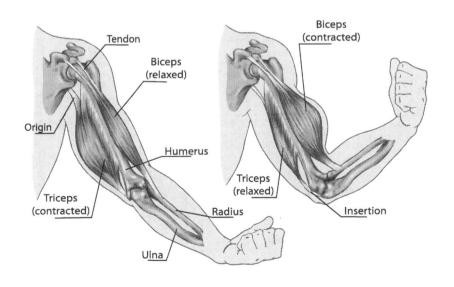

overuse injury. When a muscle contracts, the tiny myofibrils inside the muscle fibers pull together, shortening the muscle. When the muscle shortens it pulls on its tendons which then pull on the bones they are attached to. This pulling results in movement or isometrics (i.e. flexing or holding a position).

Muscles create movement by scrunching together and pulling on bones but the nervous system is what initiates muscle contraction. Nerves take messages from the brain and the spinal cord and relay them to the muscles. Once the muscle gets the message to contract, numerous biochemical reactions take place and cross-bridges scrunch protein filaments.

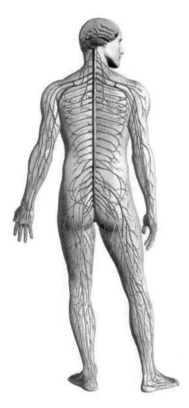

The nervous system itself is made up of two sub systems: the central nervous system (CNS) consisting of the brain and the spinal cord, and the peripheral nervous system (PNS) consisting of all the nerves throughout the body stemming from the CNS. These nerves carry signals and information throughout the body by using electrical energy called the nerve impulse (8). There are two main classifications of nerves. Sensory nerves transfer sensory perceptions such as touch, heat, pain, pressure, etc. to the CNS, creating awareness of the body's state. Motor nerves send messages the other direction, from the CNS to various locations throughout the body to initiate an action or movement.

The entire nervous system looks similar to the root system of a large tree. From the CNS, motor nerves branch out through the body and embed into muscle at what is called a neuromuscular joint or motor endplate (4,5,8,12). By branching out, one motor nerve may innervate from 1 to 500 or more muscle fibers (8). This set of one "alpha" motor nerve and all the muscle fibers it innervates is called a motor unit. Because motor units contract either completely or not at all, the number of motor units actively innervating an entire muscle determines the variability or precision that a specific muscle can have. If only 10 of 100 motor units tell their muscle fibers to contract, then a small precise movement will result. On the other hand, if 90 of the 100 motor units tell their fibers to contract, a large, powerful movement will result. The presence of multiple motor units within a muscle and their all or nothing contraction is what allows for varying levels of strength from one muscle.

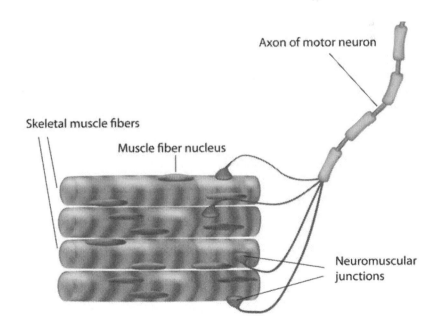

Proprioception and Flexibility

The nervous system stimulates skeletal muscles to contract but it doesn't just randomly choose muscles to stimulate. In addition to conscious direction from the central nervous system (i.e. thought), muscle stimulation is also affected by proprioception, or messages relayed to the body by various receptors that inform the body of its position, surroundings, and condition. Several of these receptors inform about sensory information, such as pressure and touch on the skin, positions, velocities, and pressures at the joints. Others, called musculotendinous receptors, sense what is happening in skeletal muscles, often inducing one or more involuntary muscular reactions.

One of the main musculotendinous receptors, called the Golgi tendon organ (GTO), is located in number in the tendons of skeletal muscle very close to where the muscle and tendon attach to each other. The main role of these receptors is to sense stretch in the tendon and to protect that tendon from the muscle pulling it apart. When a large enough stretch is sensed within the tendon, the Golgi tendon organs send a message to the central nervous system. The CNS then sends a message to the muscle to stop contracting which stops the muscles action of pulling on the tendon. In other words, when a muscle starts to pull too hard on its tendon in order to move or hold a bone, these receptors shout out a warning saying, "hey, you better stop pulling so hard or you are going to pull this tendon apart!" The nervous system then reacts by relaxing the muscle. The action of Golgi tendon organs can seem very frustrating at times during pole. For example, when holding a physically intense trick, you may come to a point where your muscles just "give in" and you fall out of the position. This happens because, as the Golgi tendon organs sense that a muscle is beginning to pull on its tendon harder than the tendon can handle, the GTO's yell out, "whoa! We are experiencing some major tension in this tendon down here! You better relax this muscle before it rips!" The nervous system then automatically relaxes the muscle and it "gives in." Despite the frustration, it's comforting to know that the action of the GTO's skillfully protects the body from crippling injury.

The other main musculotendinous receptor is called the muscle spindle or stretch receptor. These receptors are located within skeletal muscle as tiny fibers wrapped around individual muscle fibers. Like the Golgi tendon organs, muscle spindles are also sensitive to stretch but the reaction to their detection of stretch in the muscle is the opposite of GTO's. When a muscle is stretched, the spring like spindles wrapped around the fibers also stretch. Depending on the characteristics of the stretch (i.e. speed and intensity of stretch), the receptors send a message to the CNS which then may send a message for the muscle to contract in response to the stretch. This is also a protective function of the body. For example, if someone tries to stretch their hamstring too far too quickly, the muscle spindles will sense this and shout out, "ahhh!!! Our muscle is going to be pulled apart! Pull it back! Pull it back!" The central nervous system receives this message and responds by telling the muscle to contract to avoid being pulled apart. This can help protect from serious injury but it doesn't mean that great flexibility can't be obtained. When holding a stretch in a slow and controlled manner, the muscle spindles begin to relax in there "mayday" signaling to the central nervous system, and over time, a greater range of motion can be obtained as the spindles and nervous system learn that these new ranges of motion are safe.

Because Golgi tendon organs and muscle spindles have opposite reactions to stretch, they must work together in order to create the perfect balance of muscle contraction and relaxation for smooth movement. This takes intricate and complex orchestration of each proprioceptor, the nervous system, and skeletal muscles and goes to show how incredible the human body is.

In addition to muscle spindles and Golgi tendon organs, there are a few additional physiological factors that affect flexibility (1,2,8). These include skeletal structure, bony alteration, and scar tissue from past injuries, but connective tissue generally has the largest influence on flexibility and range of motion. Connective tissues, including fascia, tendons, ligaments, and muscle collagen provide adequate tensile strength to protect and bind muscle tissue and bones throughout the body. Due to these qualities, these tissues are generally less elastic and stiff. Higher concentrations of connective tissues throughout the body can be one explanation for naturally low flexibility. Thankfully, drastic increases in flexibility can be seen over time with consistent stretching and movement.

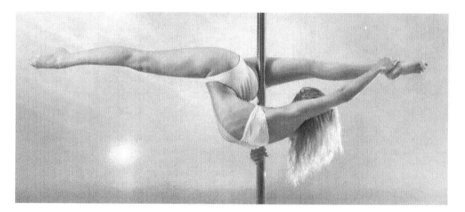

Bioenergetics

Just as a car needs fuel to move, in order for the tiny crossbridges to scrunch the small strands within the muscle fibers, and ultimately contract an entire muscle, they have to have energy. The "fuel" of the muscle is a molecule called Adenosine Triphosphate or ATP. To understand how the body gets energy from ATP, imagine holding a wood pencil with both hands. It feels strong and sturdy but when 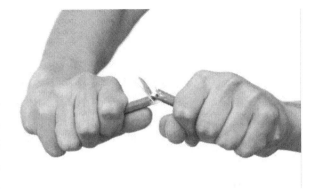 you apply pressure to both ends, it starts to bend. As you apply more pressure it finally breaks, making a loud snap, sending tiny splinters and paint flying through the air. The sound and the shards of pencil flying through the air are forms of energy. This is exactly what happens in the body. ATP is a molecule made up of four small pieces connected together with chemical bonds. When one of these bonds (the third phosphate bond) is broken, energy is released. This energy then becomes available for use by the cross-bridges, allowing them to pull Actin and Myosin together, scrunching the muscle fibers.

Most skeletal muscles only have enough ATP stored in them to provide energy for a matter of seconds, so without replenishment, most of us wouldn't even be able to make it out of bed. To keep muscles constantly supplied with ATP, the body utilizes multiple metabolic processes where molecules obtained from food go through numerous chemical reactions to reconstruct or produce new ATP molecules. These processes and their unique roles are foundational in athletic development and training program design. The two main metabolic processes used to provide ATP are probably familiar terms: Anaerobic and Aerobic metabolism. The largest difference between these two processes is the use of oxygen. During Anaerobic metabolism, oxygen is not used to reconstruct and produce new ATP molecules. Instead, anaerobic metabolism uses a combination of two different oxygen free processes to create ATP. The first of these, called the Phosphagen System, provides small amounts of energy very rapidly through the breakdown of a molecule stored within the muscle called Phosphocreatine (PC). Like the ATP molecules, when a bond in the PC molecule is broken, energy is released. During powerful, high intensity movement, the body uses this energy to put the ATP molecules back together. Once the ATP molecules are reconstructed, they are available to be broken down again to supply the muscle with more usable energy to contract. This process occurs very quickly providing high power output, but due to the limited amount of PC in the muscles, cannot be sustained for extended periods of time.

The second process in anaerobic metabolism is anaerobic glycolysis. Through this process ATP molecules are reconstituted or formed using energy created when glucose is broken down. Like ATP and PC, glucose (a sugar molecule originating from carbohydrate) is made up of smaller components held together with chemical bonds. During anaerobic glycolysis, these bonds are broken throughout a series of 12 sequential chemical reactions (all without oxygen present). The energy created from breaking these bonds during these chemical reactions is then used to form ATP. Because of the increased number of reactions that take place (as compared to the Phosphagen system), anaerobic glycolysis takes a little bit longer to form ATP but still works relatively rapidly, making it useful for higher intensity, strength and power movement. One thing to note about this system is that the breakdown of glucose during the 12 sequential chemical reactions is incomplete. The end product is lactic acid which must be further dealt with by the aerobic metabolic system. This production of lactic acid is what causes "the burn" during intense physical activity.

The Aerobic metabolic system also provides ATP energy for muscular contraction but has several key differences. The most obvious of these is that it can only take place when sufficient oxygen is available at the location of metabolism (i.e. the muscle where ATP is needed). This oxygen is required for the biochemical reactions of the aerobic system to take place. The aerobic system is also much more complicated than its anaerobic counterpart. It consists of three subsystems (aerobic glycolysis, Krebs cycle, and the electron transport system) that each consist of numerous chemical reactions and work together to produce ATP. Because of the complexity and nature of these reactions, the aerobic system is much slower than the anaerobic system but as a result, has a much higher efficiency, producing 13 to 19 times more ATP for a given amount of glucose (8). The consequence of this is the body's reliance on the aerobic system for activities that involve lower intensity, endurance exercise or movement. A final key role of the aerobic system is the breakdown of lactic acid produced by the anaerobic system. This cleanup role is conducted through chemical reactions within a subsystem of aerobic metabolism and is critical to minimize muscular fatigue and keeps the anaerobic system functioning.

The difference between anaerobic and aerobic metabolism can be illustrated with an analogy. If your car runs out of gas a few miles away from the nearest station, you will have to go get some sort of small container, fill it up with fuel, bring this to your car, dump it in the gas tank, and then use it to tentatively drive a short distance to the nearest gas station. Once you get to the gas station you'll pull up and fill your tank with fuel straight from the pump, then drive away, petal to the metal. In both cases the fuel or energy source (gasoline) was the same, but the way that the gasoline was delivered to the tank, and the way that the car performed afterward were different. Although both systems are active to some extent during exercise, anaerobic metabolism is used to create ATP during short, intense exercise lasting up to 2-3 minutes. It only uses phosphocreatine (PC) and glucose and can only produce relatively small amounts of ATP. Aerobic metabolism, on the other hand, is much more active during lower intensity, endurance exercise and primarily uses glucose and derivatives of fatty acids and amino acids (protein) to produce large volumes of ATP.

Table 2.1: Characteristics of Anaerobic and Aerobic Metabolism		
	Anaerobic Metabolism	Aerobic Metabolism
ATP Produced per mole of glucose	3 moles (anaerobic glycolysis)	39 moles
Relative Complexity	Low	High
Primary supported activity	Power, strength, intensity	Low intensity, endurance
Fuels used to create ATP	Phosphocreatine, glucose/glycogen	Glucose/glycogen, fats and protein (through secondary reactions)
Primary muscle fiber type supported	Type II	Type I

All this information may seem like trivial jargon to the athlete who is simply interested in training to achieve their performance goals, but as we will cover later, awareness of bioenergetics is critical in proper training design and can determine whether or not athletic goals are achieved.

Physiological Factors Affecting Muscular Strength

We all know intuitively that a body builder has stronger biceps than a competitive marathon runner, but what is different about the two athlete's arm muscles? The first and most obvious difference is size. Muscular hypertrophy (or size increase) is caused by an increase in muscle fiber size. As a muscle fiber increases in size, it is able to hold more myofibrils. This means that there are more tissue strands scrunching the muscle together, which results in greater force output or strength.

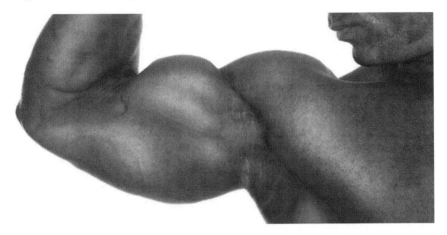

An additional, often under-credited source affecting muscular strength is the nervous system. As mentioned before, the contraction of a skeletal muscle is controlled by multiple motor nerves acting independently to activate their respective muscle fibers. It makes sense then, that if more fibers can be activated (or contracted) at one time, muscle force output (i.e. strength) will increase. This concept is referred to as multiple motor unit summation or recruitment (3,8) because the force of each muscle fiber that is activated by its motor nerve is added to the forces of all the other muscle fibers that are activated by their respective nerves.

Overall muscular strength is also affected by the frequency or timing of muscle fiber innervation (3,4,5,7,8). In order for the forces of different fibers to "add up," they must be stimulated by their nerves at the same time. This concept, called synchronization, can be understood by imagining the difference between the single small force each time one child hits a piñata 10 times versus the huge force encountered if 10 children all hit it at the same exact time. Bompa et al. state that "motor unit synchronization may exert its greatest influence on performance of activities that require the coactivation of multiple muscles at the same time (3)." Considering pole fitness often requires the use of numerous different muscles at the same time, it would make sense that this is one of the reasons sizeable strength gains are often rapidly seen in the sport.

In addition to motor unit summation and synchronization, the speed that a nerve can activate a muscle fiber over and over, called unit firing rate, affects how much total force a muscle can produce. If the nerve can get the "contract" message to the muscle fiber faster, the fiber has less time of rest in between contractions, resulting in a muscle with a greater number of contracting fibers at any given time. More contracting fibers in the muscle means greater force output.

Another variable in muscular performance is muscle fiber type. Although every skeletal muscle fiber serves the same purpose (i.e. scrunch up to provide muscular force), muscle fibers are broken down into two different general categories: Type I and Type II. Type I fibers are also known as slow twitch or slow-oxidative fibers because these fibers are superior at relatively slower but longer lasting endurance activity. Compared to Type II, Type I fibers have a slower speed of contraction but are more efficient and economical in their use of ATP (energy). They are also comparatively resistant to fatigue due largely to their use of the aerobic metabolic system, one that creates a consistent, large supply of ATP (3,4,5,8,12,13). These characteristics are ideal for postural muscles that must contract for long periods of time and athletics or movement requiring relatively low absolute strength, intensity, and speed but necessitating greater endurance capabilities, such as cross country skiing and long distance running. Athletics largely encompassing aerobic performance rely upon, exercise, and strengthen Type I fibers more than Type II.

Type II fibers are also referred to as fast-twitch or fast-glycolytic fibers due to their relatively fast speed of contraction and their reliance on anaerobic glycolysis. As opposed to Type I, Type II fibers are used for quicker, higher intensity contraction (movement or isometric contraction) and large force production. They are primarily fueled by the quick anaerobic metabolic system and therefore have much lower endurance capabilities. In other words, they are fast and strong but can't perform as long as the Type I fibers. Foss et al. also state that "the force output is much greater for Type II fibers because they wave summate [muscle fiber wave synchronization] more quickly" (8). Additionally, Type II fibers generally have a larger cross sectional area, enabling them to hold more contractile protein filaments. This results in a higher force output (8). These characteristics lead to the preferential use of Type II fibers (and the anaerobic system) in athletics requiring high intensity, strength, and speed such as sprinting, weight lifting, plyometrics, and pole fitness.

A final influence on the ability of muscles to produce strength and power is flexibility and the stretch shortening cycle (SSC). The stretch shortening cycle refers to the combination of an eccentric muscle contraction (lengthening of the muscle) followed by a concentric contraction (shortening of the muscle). This combination of muscular contractions creates additional force during the final concentric contraction due to stored elastic energy and activation of the stretch reflex (3,9). This concept is why a person usually squats down before they jump and why a baseball pitcher raises his hand above his head before he throws a ball. As flexibility increases, the ability of a muscle to lengthen or eccentrically contract is increased. The enhancement of eccentric contraction results in a boost in strength and speed during concentric muscle contraction involved in all of the pulling and pushing movements in pole.

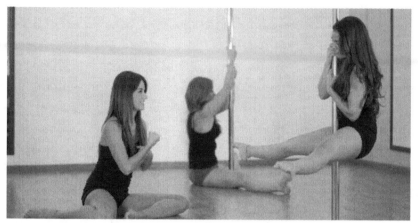

As part of the stretch shortening cycle, when a muscle is eccentrically contracted or actively lengthened (seen in the middle athlete), a more forceful concentric contraction or pull is made (seen in the athlete on the right).

Continuing Education Questions

1. What creates the pulling force inside each muscle fiber? How is this translated into overall muscle contraction?
2. How do muscles create movement?
3. What connects muscle to bone?
4. What are the two subsystems of the nervous system?
5. What is a motor unit?
6. What is the difference between a Golgi tendon organ and a muscle spindle?
7. What is the foundational "fuel" required by skeletal muscle?
8. List some of the differences between aerobic and anaerobic metabolism.
9. What are some of the physiological factors that affect strength?

References and Additional Sources

1. Allerheiligen, W. B. (1994). Stretching and warm-up. In T. R. Baechle (Ed.), Essentials of strength training and conditioning (pp. 289-313). Champaign, IL: Human Kinetics.

2. Blakey, W. P. (1994). Stretching without pain (pp. 7-35). Sechelt, B.C.: Twin Eagles Educational & Healing Institute.

3. Bompa, T. O., & Haff, G. F. (2009). Periodization: Theory and methodology of training (5th ed.). Champaign, IL: Human Kinetics.

4. Bompa, T. O., Pasquale, M. D., & Cornacchia, L. J. (2003). Serious strength training. (2nd ed.). Champaign, IL: Human Kinetics.

5. Bryant, C. X., & Green, D. J. (2010). ACE's essentials of exercise science for fitness professionals. San Diego, CA: American Council on Exercise.

6. Calais-Germain, B., & Anderson, S. (1993). Anatomy of movement. Seattle, WA: Eastland Press.

7. Dudley, G. A. (1994). Neuromuscular adaptations to conditioning. In T. R. Baechle (Ed.), Essentials of strength training and conditioning (pp. 289-313). Champaign, IL: Human Kinetics.

8. Foss, M. L., & Keteyian, S. J. (1998). Fox's physiological basis for exercise and sport. (6th ed., pp. 108-158). Boston, MA: WCB/McGraw-Hill.

9. Harman, E. (1994). The biomechanics of resistance exercise. In T. R. Baechle (Ed.), Essentials of strength training and conditioning (pp. 67-81). Champaign, IL: Human Kinetics.

10. Kapit, W., & Elson, L. M. (1993). The anatomy coloring book. New York, NY: HarperCollins College.

11. Kraemer, W. J. (1994). General adaptations to resistance and endurance training programs. In T. R. Baechle (Ed.), Essentials of strength training and conditioning (pp. 128-147). Champaign, IL: Human Kinetics.

12. Marieb, E. N., & Hoehn, K. (2010). Human anatomy & physiology. San Francisco, CA: Pearson/Benjamin Cummings.
13. Stone, M. H., & Conley, M. S. (1994). Bioenergetics. In T. R. Baechle (Ed.), Essentials of strength training and conditioning (pp. 67-81). Champaign, IL: Human Kinetics.

Chapter 3
Principles of Training

Principle of Adaptation

When it comes down to it, the foundational concept of athletic training is really quite simple. Training is a balance between stress and recovery. When our bodies experience repeated stress, they seek to adapt to better handle that stress in the future. After each bout of training (stress applied to the body), the body requires time to recover from the applied stress and return to a level of balance or homeostasis. It is during this time of recovery that the body deals with things like lactic acid build up, circulating hormone levels, restoration of energy stores, stressed muscles and tendons, and increased protein synthesis. If both the stress and recovery levels are sufficient, the training bout will result in a higher level of homeostasis and thus performance. As more bouts of training and recovery are applied, the base level of performance increases. In other words, training all comes down to the principle of adaptation. In order to protect itself and survive, the human body adapts to the conditions it experiences.

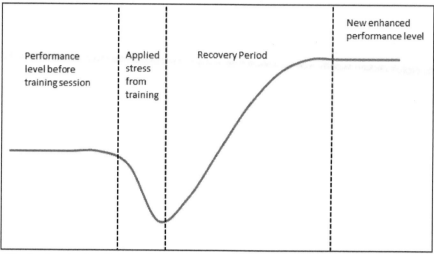

The body adapts after applied training stress and adequate recovery resulting in enhanced performance levels.

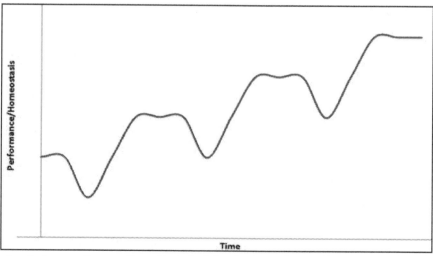

Applied correctly over time, the principle of adaptation works cumulatively to result in notable increases in performance levels.

There are, however, two situations in which the application of stress and recovery will <u>not</u> enhance performance. The first of these is when the intensity of the stress stimulus (i.e. training session) is insufficient. If the training bout is not out of the ordinary compared to what the body is used to, the body has no reason to adapt. A training program that consists of the same resistance, difficulty, movement, intensity, etc. over a long period of time will not result in a continuous increase in performance. This concept, however, should not be taken to extremes, as is often the case in popular exercise practice. The level of applied stress must be increased gradually over time in order to prevent the body from becoming overwhelmed.

In addition to inadequate amounts of applied stress, the body also fails to adapt to higher levels of performance if the amount of recovery is not sufficient. Recovery is the time in the adaptation sequence where gains in performance are actually realized. It is the time when the body compensates for the stress it underwent and prepares itself for more bouts in the future. If the body isn't given enough time, nutrients, and rest before more stress is applied, it is unable to return homeostasis. As more stress is applied, the base level of homeostasis and performance decreases. If this cycle continues, overtraining will develop. Because of its huge role in adaptation, adequate recovery is critical to increase athletic performance.

The most obvious type of stress experienced by the body in the training process is physiological stress from physical exercise. This training-induced stress results in a depletion of glycogen stores in skeletal muscles, release of multiple stress related hormones, build-up of lactic acid, and possible muscle protein catabolism (breakdown), among other things (1,2,7,11,12). Due to the body's reaction to the applied stress, it is in a temporary state of imbalance until recovery takes place. Interestingly, the physical body also reacts similarly to psychological stress. According to Keizer, "Once a stressor (physical exercise, psychic stress) has exceeded a certain threshold, a systemic reaction takes place that includes the brain and peripheral components, the HPA [hypothalamic-pituitary-adrenocortical], and the sympathetic nervous system (11)." In other words, both physical exercise and psychological stress activate a multitude of the same stress related hormones in the body. The most notable of these (in the context of stress affects) are the glucocorticoids, which can exert a catabolic (breakdown) effect on skeletal muscle when the applied stress passes a certain threshold, and sex hormones such as testosterone (7,11). Cortisol itself (one of the most important glucocorticoids) ordinarily serves as an anti-inflammatory and metabolism regulator but when the body experiences prolonged exposure to glucocorticoids due to stress, cortisol receptors within the body become less responsive. This not only decreases their ability to prevent inflammation but it also decreases Testosterone's ability to promote protein synthesis (i.e. build muscles). It also inhibits the release of growth hormone, and increases protein degradation. This is all to say that both physical and psychological stresses have a cumulative effect on the physical body. When determining the amount of stress that the body should undergo in order to induce adaptation (i.e. increase in athletic performance), it is essential that psychological stress is also accounted for.

There are several labels for the principle of adaptation in the world of athletic training including "the training effect," "supercompensation," "General Adaptive Syndrome," and "progressive overloading." Each of these theories is just a different way of explaining the principle of adaptation. They each describe different phases or categories of the rest and recovery process that complete the stress/adaptation cycle. The "supercompensation" description, as presented by Bompa et al., breaks down the principle of adaptation into four different phases that nicely describe what happens in the body throughout the process of training and adaptation (1).

Phase I of supercompensation lasts 1 to 2 hours after training begins and describes the physiological causes of fatigue experienced by the body due to the applied stress. These include lactic acid accumulation, reduction of motor unit activation, depletion of energy substrate, and delayed onset muscle soreness. Phase II begins at the onset of rest and lasts 24 to 48 hours. It is described as the compensation phase during which muscle glycogen is restored and protein synthesis rate increases. Phase III begins after 36 to 72 hours and is where the adaptation to stress is seen as a performance increase. It is characterized by the cessation of muscle soreness, the return of strength, and complete restoration of glycogen stores. Phase III is also the time when most people experience feelings of higher confidence, energy, and positive thinking. This "Psychological supercompensation" is a great indicator that

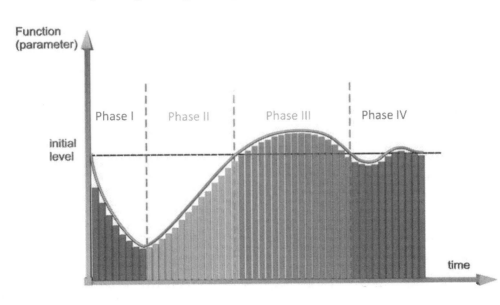

the body is ready for more training. The last phase of supercompensation, Phase IV, is the highly variable time period during which another stress stimulus (i.e. training session) should be applied before the body returns to previous homeostasis levels.

Specificity of Training

Although the principle of adaptation explains how applied stress or training results in adaptation and increased performance, it doesn't explain how different stresses or types of training result in different adaptations or changes in performance. These differences are explained by the concept of specificity of training.

To many of us this concept makes intuitive sense. If a person were to consistently lift weights with their right arm but do nothing with their left, they could only expect to see strength gains in their right arm. This is obvious because the athlete is only stressing the muscles in his right arm so it is only reasonable that these would be the only ones to adapt. We also intuitively know that a marathon runner wouldn't exercise the same as a body builder or vice versa. But why is this? To answer this question we must return to bioenergetics and muscle fiber type.

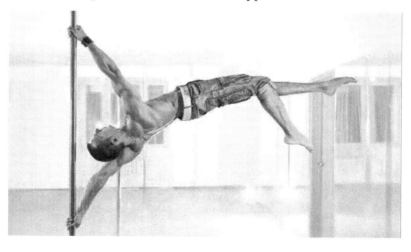

As you may recall, bioenerget-ics has to do with the way in which a muscle gets energy in order to contract, namely aero-bic or anaerobic metabolism. Depending on the activity, the body's muscles rely on each of these energy pathways in vary-ing degrees. Higher intensity, shorter duration, strength exer-cises are much more dependent on the anaerobic system while lower intensity endurance ac-tivities depend largely on the aerobic system. It makes sense 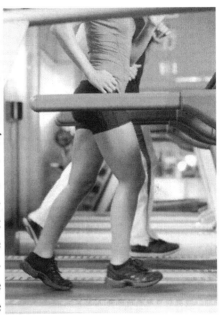 then, that the more you train a specific metabolic system, the greater performance increase you will see in the activities that that system supports. If, for example, a training program largely involves explosive, short duration exercises that call upon the an-aerobic system, then the results would be improvement in shorter duration, higher intensity performance. In contrast, a training pro-gram that focuses on the aerobic system, consisting of moderate endurance training such as jogging, would not result in improved short duration, high intensity performance. In fact, training the metabolic system opposite of that involved in the targeted sport can very readily reduce the desired performance.

In their book "Periodization: Theory and Methodology of Train-ing," Bompa et al. describe the concepts of "low-intensity exer-cise endurance (LIEE)" which characterizes aerobic training and sports involving lower intensity and greater endurance, and "high-intensity exercise endurance (HIEE)" which involves anaerobic training consisting of higher intensity, power, and strength movement (1). Along with the support of multiple scientific literature resources, Bompa et al. use the concepts of LIEE versus HIEE to emphasize the incidence of decreased anaerobic performance when aerobic training is introduced. They state "When LIEE is used to improve endurance in athletes who participate in sports that rely predominantly on anaerobic energy supply, marked decreases in power generating capacity are noted and performance is usually impaired...LIEE training can also impede muscular growth, which will impair an athlete's ability to generate high rates of force development, maximize peak force-generating capacity, and optimize peak power generation (1)." Some of the known effecters of this phenomenon are changes in motor unit recruitment, fiber type ratio shifts due to hypertrophy of individual fiber types, changes in capillary density, and cell signaling (1).

In other words, training aerobically decreases anaerobic performance. This concept is particularly relevant to pole fitness athletes as (depending on the style and skill level) pole is predominately an anaerobic activity, involving brief to intermediate bouts of intense strength and power output. This means that adding an aerobic endurance routine, such as long distance jogging, to a pole fitness training program will reduce the strength and power performance of the pole athlete (1,7).

In their contribution to the book "Overtraining in Sport," Kraemer and Nindle review multiple studies (3,4,5,6,8,9,10) to come to the same conclusion. They state that "high-intensity strength training produces a potent stimulus for muscle cell hypertrophy that appears to be mediated via increased protein synthesis and accretion of contractile proteins. Conversely, an oxidative endurance training stress causes muscle to respond in an opposite fashion by ultimately degrading and sloughing myofibril protein to optimize the kinetics of oxygen uptake (12)." In other words, the body adapts to optimize the physiological systems that are stressed.

Is this all to say that pole athletes should not participate in any aerobic fitness? You have probably heard the saying "everything in moderation." Aerobic fitness is not a complete loss in anaerobic training and does have its place depending on athletic goals, experience, and fitness level. As in any other sport, it is important that a multilateral base is developed before devoting total attention and effort to specialized training. This multilateral base, or general fitness, includes the development of endurance, strength, speed, flexibility, and coordination and requires both anaerobic and aerobic training (1). For a person just beginning their pole fitness journey, a portion of aerobic training in addition to the distinct anaerobic portions of pole would probably serve them well. This is actually very convenient considering most beginner pole classes begin by teaching things like floor work, dance, and transitions. These more aerobic focused activities can then be built upon with a transition into more anaerobic powered movement such as spins, climbs and holds.

More advanced athletes or those with focused goals of becoming a superior pole athlete should not place any emphasis on aerobic training. Even with an intense sport such as pole, the aerobic metabolic system is always active to some degree and will receive sufficient attention throughout pole and other daily life activity. The extent to which each system is contributing to energy production depends on factors including the type and intensity of training or activity being conducted, the physiological status of the athlete, and diet.

The aerobic system makes some important contributions during anaerobically dominated activity. As mentioned in the bioenergetics section, one of these contributions is the buffering of lactic acid in the blood. This "clean-up" function of the aerobic system occurs during periods of rest from anaerobic glycolysis and is critical in preparing the body for additional bouts of anaerobic exercise. Aerobic metabolism also provides critical energy during lower intensity movement interspersed with higher intensity and supplies energy to crucial postural muscles and organs. For these reasons, it may be beneficial for the serious pole athlete to support the function of the aerobic system through participation in a minor amount of aerobic activity. Note that this is different than recommending aerobic training which would involve significant and consistent aerobic exercise (i.e. jogging, elliptical, spin class, etc.) aimed at adaptation of the aerobic system. Choosing activities that are enjoyable and meaningful is a great way to obtain sufficient periodic aerobic exercise for the serious pole athlete. Activities like these, in fact, are already frequently practiced within pole training (i.e. dancing, floor work, transitions, etc.) and throughout daily life.

Finally, if your goal is to just obtain a good level of general fitness and you enjoy both pole and aerobic exercise, then go for it. The combination of these is a great way to establish a high level of multilateral development.

Continuing Education Questions

1. What are the two main components of an athletic training program?
2. What are the two situations where the application of training stress will not result in performance enhancement?
3. Is physical stress the only factor to consider when determining stress load? Why or why not?
4. During what phase of supercompensation should another training stress be applied? What are the characteristics of this phase?
5. Draw a simple curve demonstrating the principle of adaptation.

6. What types of exercise or sports rely predominantly on the anaerobic metabolic system? Aerobic system?

7. Should an athlete training for a sport dominated by anaerobic performance train aerobically? Why or why not?

References and Additional Sources

1. Bompa, T. O., & Haff, C. G. (2009). Periodization: Theory and methodology of training (5th ed.). Champaign, IL: Human Kinetics.

2. Bompa, T. O., Cornacchia, L. J., & Pasquale, M. P. (2003). Serious strength training (2nd ed., pp. 3-20). Champaign, IL: Human Kinetics.

3. Chromiak, J. A., & Mulvaney, D. R. (1990). A Review: The Effects of Combined Strength and Endurance Training on Strength Development. The Journal of Strength and Conditioning Research, 4(2), 55-60. doi: 10.1519/1533-4287(1990)0042.3.CO;2

4. Deschenes, M. R., Maresh, C. M., Crivello, J. F., Armstrong, L. E., Kraemer, W. J., & Covault, J. (1993). The effects of exercise training of different intensities on neuromuscular junction morphology. Journal of Neurocytology, (22), 603-615.

5. Dudley, G. A., & Djamil, R. (1985). Incompatibility of endurance and strength training modes of exercise. Journal of Applied Physiology, (59), 1446-1451.

6. Dudley, G. A., & Fleck, S. J. (1987). Strength and endurance training: Are they mutually exclusive? Sports Medicine, (4), 79-85.

7. Foss, M. L., & Keteyian, S. J. (1998). Fox's physiological basis for exercise and sport. (6th ed.). Boston, MA: WCB/McGraw-Hill.

8. Hennessy, L. C., & Watson, A. W. (1994). The Interference Effects of Training for Strength and Endurance Simultaneous-

ly. The Journal of Strength and Conditioning Research, 8(1), 12-19. doi: 10.1519/1533-4287(1994)0082.3.CO;2

9. Hickson, R. C. (1980). Interference of strength development by simultaneously training for strength and endurance. European Journal of Applied Sport Science Research, (45), 255-269.

10. Hunter, G., Demment, R., & Miller, P. (1987). Development of strength and maximum oxygen uptake during simultaneous training for strenth and endurance. Journal of Sports Medicine and Physical Fitness, (27), 269-275.

11. Keizer, H. A. (1998). Neuroendocrine aspects of overtraining. In R. B. Kreider, A. C. Fry, & M. L. O'Toole (Eds.), Overtraining in sport (pp. 145-159). Champaign, IL: Human Kinetics.

12. Kraemer, W. J., & Nindl, B. C. (1998). Factors involved with overtraining for strength and power. In R. B. Kreider, A. C. Fry, & M. L. O'Toole (Eds.), Overtraining in sport (pp. 69-86). Champaign, IL: Human Kinetics.

13. Wathen, D., & Roll, F. (1994). Training methods and modes. In T. R. Baechle (Ed.), Essentials of strength training and conditioning (pp. 403-414). Champaign, IL: Human Kinetics.

14. Wathen, D. (1994). Periodization: Concepts and applications. In T. R. Baechle (Ed.), Essentials of strength training and conditioning (pp. 459-472). Champaign, IL: Human Kinetics.

Chapter 4
Overtraining

Definition of Overtraining

As discussed before, increases in performance through training occur when stress is applied and followed by an adequate recovery period. When the body is consistently unable to fully recover from training bouts, it enters into what is called a state of overtraining. The term "overtraining" can be somewhat confusing because it not only encompasses a process but an outcome as well. When an athlete consistently does not obtain an adequate amount of recovery because of training volumes, non-training stress, and a lack of rest, they are in the process of overtraining. This process then leads to physiological, psychological, and performance decrements which are often themselves referred to as overtraining, overtraining symptoms, or "overtraining syndrome." In addition, numerous other terms have been used to describe the process and outcome of stress and recovery imbalance. These include staleness, burnout, overfatigue, overwork, overload, under-performance, under-recovery, and overtraining behavior (5,23,37,38). These are all used in an attempt to pin down in one phrase exactly what a stress imbalance in the body is. Unfortunately, the process and effects of these imbalances are highly varied from individual to individual and sport to sport. For our purposes, we will use the all-encompassing and intuitively obvious term "overtraining" to describe the process and outcomes of consistently not obtaining sufficient amounts of recovery from applied stress to the body.

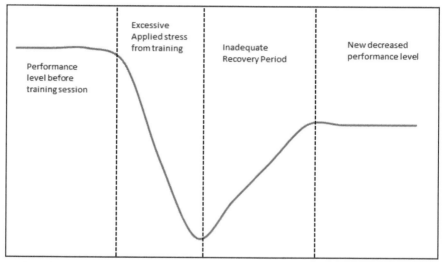

When the recovery period is not adequate, performance level decreases. Perpetuated over time, this results in symptoms of overtraining.

Prevalence and Significance in Pole

Because of the wide variations in sports, training methodology, and individual physiology and psychology, as well as differences in definitions, symptoms, causes, and degrees of overtraining, it is very difficult to determine the prevalence of overtraining in athletics or individual training. Bompa reports that symptoms of overtraining are seen in 7%-20% of elite athletes (5) while Gould et al. noted that 28% of 296 U.S. Olympians at the Atlanta games were overtrained (11). Numbers from other studies range from 5-10% up to 64% (16,29,31,34,37). If anything, it is most likely that the prevalence of overtraining is underestimated in both elite and amateur athletes. This is due in part to a lack of scientifically based training knowledge and the many misconceptions and messages conveyed about training in today's society. As mentioned in the beginning of this book, society generally supports an emotionally and physically abusive athletic and training environment with messages such as "no pain, no gain." We seem to live in a world where injury and pain are seen as badges of honor and designation of true athleticism. This environment, as will be discussed further, encourages individuals who don't know any better to train too much and rest too little. It makes sense then, that the further permeation of these messages would result in higher levels of overtraining.

As a newly developing sport, pole fitness is in a wonderful position to create a well-informed, encouraging environment that values recovery just as much as exercise. Creating this atmosphere in the pole community is especially important due to the high intensity, anaerobic nature of the sport. Even though it is fun, the training load involved in advanced pole training can be substantial, on par with and even larger than what most would consider a demanding traditional workout. Many strength training programs, for example, are designed with weight loads around 70-80% of one rep max (1RM: the maximum amount the athlete can successfully lift one time). Because pole requires the athlete to lift and hold their entire body weight, they are often training at and easily beyond 80% of 1RM for the majority of their pole session. In order to avoid overtraining then, the recovery period must reflect the need to compensate for this high intensity.

Factors Leading to Overtraining

- **Lack of recovery time**

Overtraining results when an imbalance between stress and recovery in the body develops. This imbalance can be caused by a number of different factors. The most fundamental of these is a lack of recovery time. When the body doesn't have enough time to recover, stress begins to accumulate, ultimately resulting in a steady decrease in performance. As mentioned before, both applied physical stress and psychological stress affect the physiological body in multiple ways. The body can literally be "torn down" during training through a large release of glucocorticoids (protein catabolism/breakdown), strain on muscle fibers, tendons, and bones, wear on joints, energy depletion (glycogen and phosphocreatine), and buildup of lactic acid. Without adequate recovery time, these effects of stress don't go away. Unfortunately, just like a rolling snowball, they build upon each other with the additional application of stress.

Possibly one of the most difficult things about pole is resting. It is such a fun and exciting sport in which performance gains are seen very quickly. It can be so hard to rest from poling when accomplishments are made and previously difficult moves are just within reach. It's so hard to stop for recovery time when you want to get better as fast as possible. It is absolutely critical, however, that recovery time is adequate. Otherwise, you won't get better at all. Marathon runner and athletic trainer Sage Rountree reminds us of this important point in her book The Athlete's Guide to Recovery. "You need to trust that time off, even though it might be hard to take, will have a direct, positive effect on your training (38)."

- **Training volume/intensity**

As O'Toole states, "The ideal [training] adaptation results from being able to manipulate the combination of volume and intensity in the correct ratio of work to rest (32)." It makes sense then, that excessive training volume and intensity can also be major contributors to overtraining in athletes. Prolonged high training volume and intensity disturb the stress/recovery cycle in the same way that a lack of recovery time does. In addition, they can decrease resting testosterone concentrations which in turn reduces protein synthesis (muscle building) and increase resting cortisol levels which can lead to an increase in protein catabolism (muscle degradation) (7,17,43). This is not to say that high levels of training volume and intensity are never warranted. These in fact can be beneficial to a performance enhancing training program. The key to productive training is that high levels are not consistently sustained without adequate rest.

In our society it is often hard to know how much is too much. Our bodies may be telling us one thing but the common message is that more is always better. Apart from a periodized and intuitive training program, as will be discussed later, a study by A.C. Fry et. al gives a good perspective on the shockingly relative ease that overtraining can be induced with what our society would most likely consider a low training volume (8,9).

In their study, individuals participated in a training session six days per week for two weeks. The session consisted of 10 repetitions of a squat exercise on a squat simulating machine (i.e. Smith Machine) at a resistance as close to their 1 rep max (1 RM) as possible at that given time. After each squat, the individual rested for two minutes. In other words, each participant did 10 squats per day for 12 days (with two rest days during the study) with the most weight that they could successfully lift. Although it doesn't seem to be a whole lot compared to what we are often "told" we should do, this program elicited obvious overtraining symptoms seen by strength decrements of >10% reduction in 1RM strength and a 2-8 week period after the study before any of the participants were able to resume a normal lower body strength routine. It's also interesting to note that strength decrements were also seen in low velocity knee extension showing that the overtraining syndrome even affected other types of movement in addition to the squat.

This study goes to show that the volume and intensities that are often communicated as good athletic practice may very well lead to a state of overtraining syndrome. It is important to be cognizant of the stress/recovery balance on an individual basis. Elevated training volumes and intensity will stress each body differently. Too much too hard will result in strength and performance decrements, sometimes lasting weeks to months.

The rate at which training volume and intensity are increased is also an important consideration. According to Kraemer and Nindl, "The most common mistake made in training is most likely related to the rate of progression. If mechanical and chemical loads are created which damage the fundamental morphological structures involved with the adaptational changes (e.g. increased muscle size) required for improved performance, overtraining can occur rapidly (20)." In other words, do too much too fast, and your likely to burn out or get hurt very quickly.

- **Lack of individualization**

One of the nifty things about cooking and baking is that nearly anyone with a recipe and a decent ability to measure can reproduce dishes nearly identical to anyone else using the same recipe. This makes sense. You put the same things in and you get the same things out. Unfortunately, training is not like cooking. The same training program applied to two different people will almost never result in the same changes in performance. This is not only due to the myriad of physiological differences from person to person, but is also due to differences in things such as training background and experience, health status, level of multilateral development, diet, and social and psychological stress. These and the other factors listed in Table 4.1 have a profound effect on the stress/recovery balance of the individual.

Table 4.1: Factors Affecting Individual Response to Applied Training Stress
• Level of multilateral development (general fitness level)
• Level of physiological homeostasis
• Physiological make-up
• Genetic potential
• Level of athletic technique
• Previous injuries
• Recovery rate
• Neuroendocrine system response (hormone response)
• Health status
• Presence of overtraining symptoms
• Biological rhythms
• Diet
• Sleep patterns
• Individual work capacity
• Social stressors
• Psychological state
• Ability to cope with external stressors
• Beliefs about the self and world
• Expectations
• Motivational goals
• Self-evaluation/perception

When the same training program is "prescribed" to a group of athletes, the individual performance outcomes will vary. Some participants may not be stressed enough to elicit possible performance gains while others may be overstressed and develop signs of overtraining. As Rowbottom et al. state "Optimal performance can only be achieved by the precise balance, on an individual basis, of training stress and adequate recovery (16)."

An interesting point is that even when athletes with similar abilities and training level are exposed to identical training programs, their performance outcomes can still vary tremendously. This could be due, for example, to psychological stress invading the life of one of the athletes. Perhaps one of them is dealing with a pending divorce, a possible layoff, or a big presentation at work. These psychosocial factors cause stress in the body, and as we know, stress in cumulative, and when stress outweighs recovery for a long enough time, performance is adversely affected.

An especially detrimental, but very tempting training practice is to mimic the training programs of elite athletes. It is tempting because intuitively, it seems that if an amateur trains the same way as a professional, they should get the same results. It is detrimental, however, because elite athletes have, over time, obtained a very elevated state of physiological homeostasis. They are able to withstand much higher stress levels for a given amount of rest without experiencing symptoms of overtraining. In fact, these athletes require higher levels of stress to maintain or increase their current levels of homeostasis. If an amateur athlete adheres to a program practiced by a professional, they are very likely to experience damaging symptoms of overtraining, as their body will be unable to recover from the huge jump in the stress experienced.

Unfortunately, our society is often bombarded by quick fix, prescription exercise programs aimed at individuals who honestly want to improve performance but don't have the knowledge to design their own training program. It is no wonder why there are so many different books that demand specific training regimens. Each new one that comes out never quite seems to result in the performance outcomes that it advertised. These exercise "cookbooks" can't account for all of the differences from person to person and therefore, cannot produce consistent results. Instead, they often leave an athlete undertrained and stagnant, or overtrained and out of commission. An optimal training program must be individualized in order to realize the most efficient and maximum performance gains while at the same time avoiding a state of overtraining.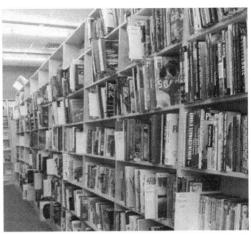

- **Monotonous training**

Just as a well-designed training program requires the correct proportion of stress and recovery, it also demands balance between repetition and variation. In order for the body to adapt, it must experience a specific stress often enough to warrant change, but if the same stresses are applied over an extended period of time, the body's need and ability to adapt is diminished. This can result in monotonous program overtraining, characterized by stagnation or decreased performance, fatigue, and/or overuse injuries (5,15,32,46). Monotonous training occurs when an athlete's exercise patterns remain the same from week to week and month to month. Although the athlete may be applying stress to their muscles, this type of training does not sufficiently stimulate the nervous system to induce additional physiological adaptation and performance gains. After time, the central nervous system becomes over adapted to the non-varying motor patterns of a repetitive program. This is why large performance gains are often seen at the beginning of a training program and stagnation seen as the same program is continued over time.

Training without variation over time can also cause disproportional wear and tear on the body. Joints are particularly susceptible to monotonous training damage. Articulating joints (called synovial joints) consist of two bones held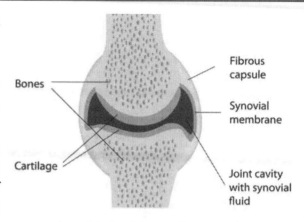

together with ligaments and padded with cartilage and a capsule of synovial fluid. With excessive and repetitive use, the cartilage and ligaments can become worn and damaged, permanently impairing the joint. Skeletal muscle, bone, and tendons are also at risk for injury. Without adequate variation, the specific body parts stressed aren't ever given the chance to fully recover.

- **Cultural demands**

Although cultural demands themselves do not force an athlete into an overtrained state, they are perhaps the strongest drivers behind the training practices that lead to maladaptation and overtraining. Many cultural messages and athletic environments create enormous amounts of guilt in an athlete. Maxims such as "no pain, no gain" and "more is better" combined with the message that the only acceptable athlete is the superior athlete, create an impossible situation for a person to train in. No one can win under these circumstances. The guilt that develops from never being able to add up combined with the inaccurate training methods and sole emphasis on stress application (exercise), can easily lead to a state of overtraining.

In an effort to keep up with cultural demands, athletes often employ an attitude of "mental toughness." This is essentially a numbing of messages from the body in order to train more and/or harder. High levels of pain and stress are tolerated and any discomfort or fatigue is pushed aside as the athlete drives on. Unfortunately, as stated by sports psychologist Dr. Trisha Leahy, "The problem with the mental toughness concept is that it implies a 'head down go as hard as you can and close off everything to reach the desired end' type of approach. It's a problematic and simplistic concept. (37)" This disassociation from important physiological indicators is a huge driver in overtraining but is still often glorified as a characteristic of "true, elite" athletes. As Dr. Leahy states, "you're a hero if your leg is broken and you can go out there and win the game for your team (37)."

- **Competitive environments**

In a culture where winning is often of the utmost importance, competitive environments are frequently precipitators of overtraining. Whether it be due to a naturally competitive personality, expectations of others, organized team or individual sports where winning is crucial for the security of the team or athlete, or rewards associated with success, a competitive atmosphere combined 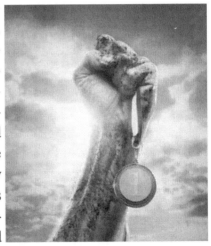 with cultural messages such as "you get what you sweat for" can encourage an athlete to train with higher volumes and intensities than their body can handle. Because recovery is often not emphasized as an important factor in improving athletic performance, it often gets neglected in an effort to beat the next competitor. Unfortunately, as we have seen, this type of training typically results in the exact opposite. This is not to say that a competitive environment itself is a bad thing. A healthy level of competition can provide encouragement and purpose to a training athlete and sport. It is when the competition becomes so important that athletes begin to loose site of the importance of recovery that it becomes a major problem.

- **Guilt about not working hard enough**

Many athletes and recreational exercisers are also led to overtrain through guilt about not working hard enough. As mentioned before, cultural imperatives and maxims have created an atmosphere where more is always better. So, no matter how much an athlete does, it's never quite enough. We as consumers are bombarded with photo shopped pictures and exercise prescriptions constantly reminding us that we "should" be doing more. What is particularly interesting about this hard work guilt is that it is often even present in highly successful athletes. As Richardson et al. state, "no matter how well certain athletes perform, it is not good enough because it is not perfect (37)." They go further to say "even the experience of success can be a risk factor for overtraining...sometimes performance peaks motivate athletes to try even harder (37)." So, even when the performance goal is achieved, athletes still often feel that they should work harder. Unfortunately, their drive and the cultural imperatives that perhaps brought them their athletic success, can ultimately become their demise.

Internal stressors and psychosocial issues also fuel guilt about not working hard enough. Athletes who have lived through chaotic, unloving, or unaccepting environments may feel that superior athletic performance is the only way that they can be accepted or maintain control of their lives (27,37). When they feel unloved, anxious, out of control, or distressed, they equate these feelings with not training hard enough because training is the medium they've used to numb these feelings. When these internal stressors flare up, they are accompanied with a sense of guilt for not working hard enough to control them. Regrettably, this can be one of the most powerful and harmful drivers of overtraining because no matter how much a person stresses their body, they still experience the emotional pain associated with their past and present. In an effort to subside the pain and guilt, an athlete can easily run themselves into the ground.

- **Guilt from witnessing superior athletic performance**

Seeing another athlete perform can be a very inspiring and positive experience for some. For others, it can generate feelings of inadequacy and guilt. Not being able to perform at the same level as another, even if they are a professional, can make an athlete feel like they must be doing something wrong or that they aren't working hard enough. As stated by Richardson et al., "Athletes might find that the presence of more experienced or talented athletes can create overwhelming stress…For some this added pressure may lead to pushing excessively in training in an effort to compensate for perceived shortcomings (37)." Even with an experienced athlete, obvious explanations for differences in performance ability, such as training history, external stressors, and individual work capacity, can be completely forgotten or dismissed. The guilt that results from feeling inadequate can surpass all reason and turn spectating into an experience that fuels overtraining in an attempt to increase performance too quickly.

This potential overtraining driver is especially relevant in pole fitness, where jaw dropping performances are the hallmark of pole gatherings. Pole is a quickly developing sport with athletes participating from a range of different athletic backgrounds and abilities. There is a real danger of new pole athletes becoming overtrained in an effort to replicate the performance and athletic abilities of seasoned athletes. A message of patience and accurate training knowledge is critical in preventing overtraining and burn-out in less experienced polers.

- **Responses to poor performance**

The reason behind a maladaptive response to poor performance (i.e. adding too much training) can be summarized by a quote from an interview conducted by Richardson et al: "Train, get better. How can I train and get worse? So I'll just train harder and I'll get better (37)." As has been discussed, it is commonly believed and portrayed that the key to improving performance is more training. It makes sense then, that when an athlete underperforms (either literally or perceived), their response would be to increase their training load. As we have seen, however, performance gains don't work that way. The body requires a balance between stress and recovery in order for those gains to be realized. Training harder because of performance shortcomings only serves to speed up the process of overtraining. Soon the athlete is trapped in a downward spiral of decreased performance followed by increased training loads. This results in overtraining and further decreased performance.

- **Inadequate energy balance**

As mentioned before, ATP is the chemical compound used by the body to supply energy for muscle contraction. ATP itself is produced with energy provided by chemical compounds that the body gets from food. The body's preferred fuel, glucose, is a simple sugar converted from carbohydrate by the body. Glucose can either be immediately used to create ATP by one of the metabolic systems, stored as glycogen in the liver or skeletal muscle to be used later, or converted to fatty acids and stored as adipose tissue (body fat). Lipids (fatty acids stored in the body and fat consumed from food) are another source of energy to create ATP. Fatty acids (common lipids) provide more energy compared to the same amount of glucose but require additional steps to be metabolized as discussed below. The final dietary source of possible energy for ATP synthesis is amino acids (protein). Protein's main role in the body is muscle, tissue, and enzyme synthesis. It is the building block of the body so understandably, the body generally tends to use it in low quantities for energy production.

The body's preference in what fuel source it uses is determined by the intensity and duration of activity as these govern the relative demands on the anaerobic and aerobic metabolic systems. During high intensity, power activities, the anaerobic system is the dominant energy provider while lower intensity, endurance activities obtain a large portion of their required energy from the aerobic system. As seen in Table 4.2 on the next page, each of these metabolic systems and their subsystems can only operate on specific fuels (ultimately obtained from food). The consequences of this is that if these fuels are not available, the effected metabolic system will not be able to function optimally, and if a specific metabolic system cannot function, energy cannot be provided for the activities specific to that system. This concept is similar to the idea of diesel versus unleaded fuel at a service station. If your car is designed to run off of unleaded gasoline but you fill it up with diesel, the car will shortly quit running because it cannot operate correctly by burning diesel fuel.

A couple of interesting notes from the table are that glucose is the only fuel that can be used during both anaerobic and aerobic glycolysis. Fat and protein are only used during the Krebs Cycle (a subsystem of aerobic metabolism) and require extra preparation before their use. Since glucose is the only fuel that can be used during both anaerobic and aerobic glycolysis (7,25,42,45), what happens when carbohydrate intake isn't adequate to meet the energy demands placed on the body? The body does have one more option to try and keep things going. When glucose levels are low, the body can take amino acids from the blood, liver, or muscle tissue, and send them to the liver where they are converted to glucose through a process called gluconeogenesis. If both glucose and amino acid (protein) reserves are depleted in the blood and liver, the body is forced to use a portion of its muscle tissue in order to produce usable energy required by anaerobic and aerobic glycolysis.

Table 4.2: Fuel Sources of Metabolic Systems	
	Fuel Source
Anaerobic System	
Phosphagen System	Phosphocreatine
Anaerobic Glycolysis	Glucose
Aerobic System	
Aerobic Glycolysis	Glucose
Krebs Cycle	Glycolysis byproducts, fat after Beta Oxidation, protein after deamination
Electron Transport System	Glycolysis and Krebs Cycle byproducts

These points are critical for high intensity power sports like pole fitness, where performance is highly dependent on the fast acting anaerobic metabolic system. This system consists only of the phosphagen system and anaerobic glycolysis, neither of which can use protein or fat as direct fuel sources. If carbohydrate consumption or glycogen stores in the muscle are not adequate, anaerobic glycolysis will not be able to keep up with the intense demands of these sports. If this energy imbalance is sustained, muscle wasting and premature, long lasting fatigue will result (4,5,7,22,40).

Here is another way to picture these concepts. Imagine a home in a very frigid environment that relies on a wood burning stove for

heat. If the home own-
er keeps enough wood
on hand and continues
to feed it into the fire,
the house stays warm.
However, if the owner
runs out of firewood,
he will have to start
burning something
else or the fire will go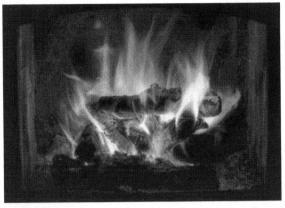
out and the house will freeze. His next option may be a stack of
old newspapers and magazines or other burnable material, but the
stove isn't designed for these so they are not going to be able to
keep up with the heat demands for very long. Pretty soon, if the
owner doesn't go get firewood, he is going to have to literally
start cutting pieces of wood off of his house so that he can keep
the fire going. In this case he has to sacrifice part of his house to
keep the rest of it from freezing. The longer he goes without real
firewood, the more and more degraded and inefficient his house
becomes.

When the body doesn't have enough glucose derived from carbohydrate (either glucose in the blood or glycogen stored in skeletal
muscle and the liver) the body will be forced to use its own building blocks, protein, as a fuel source. This process is often termed
"muscle wasting" because the body is literally "burning" portions
of itself for fuel. Over time this process results in fatigue, strength
and speed reduction, and performance decline.

In extreme cases, the perpetuation of inadequate food intake and
muscle catabolism can lead to Amenorrhea (loss of menstrual period) and Osteoporosis in women. Disordered eating and these
two conditions together are referred to as the "female athlete tri-

ad" and can have devastating effects not only on performance but on longevity of life (4,44).

• Overuse of nonsteroidal anti-inflammatory drugs

As a result of applied stress through training, micro tissues such as muscle cells and fibers within the body are often damaged, resulting in soreness and inflammation. This response is part 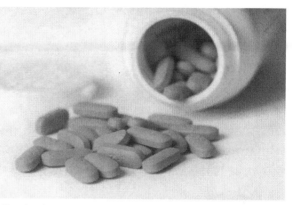 of the reason for the dip in homeostasis and performance after a training session. From time to time, nonsteroidal anti-inflammatory drugs (NSAIDs) such as ibuprofen can be taken to relieve some of the discomfort associated with these stress responses or to promote healing of a tendon injury by reducing inflammation. Problems begin to develop, however, when NSAIDs are taken too often.

In a properly designed training program, the only time a person would experience situations in which they may want to take NSAIDs would be after a rare and particularly strenuous application of stress (i.e. the training session) or after an injury is sustained. If anti-inflammatories are consistently taken in an effort to minimize recovery time, a false sense of restoration may develop, leading to the premature application of another training bout. If this cycle is continued, a larger and larger disparity in the stress/recovery balance will develop and lead to overtraining.

In addition to creating a downward spiral in the stress/recovery balance, taking NSAIDs too often can also reduce the body's ability to adapt after training (2,5,47). Despite using them in an effort to speed and enhance recovery, overuse of NSAIDs actually slows the healing process and reduces the production of myofibril proteins (12). Since these are the components of muscle fibers that do all the pulling, a reduced production of myofibrils would result in strength gain stagnation. A laboratory study conducted on rats also showed that high levels of NSAID use inhibited resistance training induced muscle hypertrophy and protein synthesis (41).

The consequences of these findings are important for the pole athlete. If NSAIDs are taken too often, strength gains will stagnate and recovery time will increase. If the use of NSAIDs is continued or even increased in order to attempt to compensate for the increased recovery time, tissue damage and soreness can be intensified. If the answer to these physiological reactions is more drugs, a devastating snowball effect will develop as the body falls further and further behind in adapting to the stresses it experiences. As it falls behind, performance will decrease and overtraining will gain more and more of a foothold on the athlete.

Outcomes of Overtraining

There are numerous possible outcomes of overtraining but the hallmark symptom and the one commonly used to diagnose overtraining is a consistent decrease in athletic performance. There are numerous overtraining outcomes that can affect performance. Training too much, too hard can have damaging physiological and psychological consequences that make it difficult or even impossible for an athlete to perform at previously attainable levels. A decrease in performance can also be seen in athletes without other obvious overtraining symptomsj simply due to accumulated fatigue.

All of the outcomes of overtraining are counter to the entire purpose of athletic training. As Bompa states, "Training is a process by which an athlete is prepared for the highest level of performance possible...the intent is to increase the athlete's skills and work capacity to optimize athletic performance (5)." Overtraining does not do this. Working too much, too hard, without adequate recovery decreases performance. Doing too much is worse than not doing anything at all. So much for the popular belief that working out harder and longer will always produce better results!

- **Accumulated fatigue and overtraining perpetuation**

Many times an athlete first experiences an overtraining induced decrease in performance without the presence of other more obvious symptoms (i.e. physical injury, high resting heart rate, depressed mood, etc.). This circumstance is simply a consequence of the principle of adaptation. If stress is consistently applied to the body before it is able to recover, fatigue accumulates, gradually diminishing the body's base performance abilities (homeostasis).

A state of accumulated fatigue can be a very dangerous place for an athlete to be. Without obvious physical signs of overtraining, an athlete may be led to train even more in an effort to compensate for their performance decline. Unfortunately for them, accumulated fatigue only goes away with rest and recovery. By adding additional stress through more training, the overtrained athlete is only accelerating their current decrease in performance and becoming more and more vulnerable to more harmful overtraining consequences. In a society where more training is nearly always the answer to poor athletic performance, the development of perpetual overtraining is alarmingly likely.

Perpetual overtraining can be described by the "snowball effect."

When a snowball first starts rolling down a hill it's usually relatively small and slow moving. With each turn it makes, however, more snow is stuck to its sides. As more snow sticks, the ball gets heavier and as the ball gets heavier, it rolls down the hill faster. As the ball rolls faster, more snow sticks to it faster. It gets bigger and bigger, faster and faster until it is barreling down the hill, totally out of control.

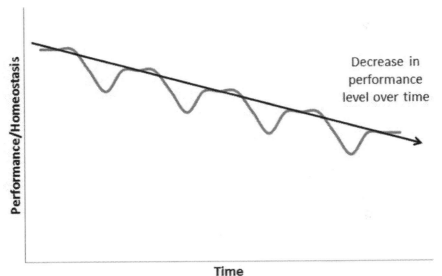

Performance decreases over time with the accumulation of fatigue.

When an athlete sees their performance levels slipping and they react by increasing training loads, they are simply "adding more snow to their snowball." When more stress is added, fatigue continues to increase. This increase in fatigue further decreases performance which may then lead the athlete to increase training loads even further. With continued decreases in performance, the athlete may start to feel desperate and become even more unreasonable as they grasp for anyway to boost their performance without resting. Their perpetuation of exercise and performance decrements begin to resemble the uncontrollable snowball, barreling down the hill.

- **Injury: musculoskeletal and orthopedic damage**

As overtraining gains a foothold, athletes become more and more susceptible to serious, long lasting consequences. Some athletes may develop the idea that they can put up with the stresses of perpetual overtraining because they've gotten away with it before. But, as stated by Richardson, "It's like a game of Russian roulette; eventually you are going to cop one with a bullet (37)."

The "bullet" that Richardson is referring to is injury. Training results in disruptions in homeostasis at the cellular level. These disruptions are a normal part of the principle of adaptation, but when adequate recovery is not allowed, typical microtraumatic damage to muscle fibers can lead to musculotendinous injury (injury of the muscles and or tendons) and reduced athletic function (19). Sometimes an acute injury is experienced by athletes (i.e. concussion, high impact or traumatic fractures, etc.) but a large majority of sports injuries are due to the cumulative effects of repeated minor injuries, muscle imbalances, weakness, fatigue, inflexibility, and inflammation, often precipitated by overtraining (5,19,37,38). In addition, the increased fatigue of an overtrained, injured musculotendinous system can lead to other bodily injuries such as stress fractures. This occurs when applied forces are transferred to supporting parts of the body because the primary muscles and tendons are no longer able to withstand them.

Athletic injury is a particularly harmful and devastating component of overtraining because it is so easily perpetuated and long lasting. Kibler and Chandler describe the development and perpetuation of overtraining injuries as a vicious cycle. "The cycle begins with localized pain that has a secondary effect of inhibiting muscle action. Repeated minor injuries, secondary to contracture, tightness, weakness, imbalance, and inflammation have a cumulative effect resulting in a chronic injury...If not completely rehabilitated, or if the athlete is allowed to return to stressful activity too early, their injury can become a chronic problem, limiting performance for an extended period of time (19)." Unfortunately, many athletes have experienced this phenomenon first hand. A pole athlete, for example, who consistently trains too hard, may slowly develop rotator cuff tendinitis in their shoulder. If they continue to train, the tendinitis will continue to get worse to the point of dehabilitation.

If they rest but return to previous training levels too soon, the injury will return and the athlete will once again be out of commission. If the athlete doesn't recognize the cycle of injury perpetuation but instead tries to train through it, they will only experience continued, worsening injury and disappointing athletic performance. Oftentimes this perpetuation results in permanent damage to the body.

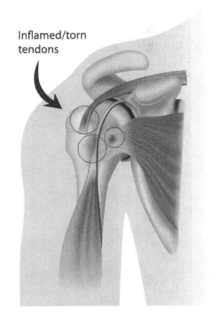

Inflamed/torn tendons

An athlete can even become caught up in the development and/or perpetuation of an overuse injury without extreme training loads. When muscles and tendons are weakened and fatigued through training, what used to be a normal load becomes a relative overload. The athlete may assume that since they are performing tasks or training routines that they normally do, they are safe from overtraining injury. Unfortunately, to a fatigued muscle, the normal load now feels like an extreme load and can damage muscles and tendons just as easily as a heavy load on rested muscles and tendons (19,24,37). This vulnerability of fatigued or previously injured tissue is one of the main reasons a slow re-entry into training is important after injury recovery.

Table 4.3: Common Repetitive Use Injuries in Pole Fitness	
Injury	Description
Rotator Cuff Tendinitis	Inflammation or injury to the rotator cuff muscles. These muscles (supraspinatus, infraspinatus, subcapularis, and teres minor) have the primary function of holding the humeral head (arm bone) in the glenoid fossa (shoulder socket).
Medial Epicondylitis	Inflammation of the wrist flexors at the medial epicondyle (inside of the elbow). Usually caused by force overload with pain most noticeable during use. Also known as Golfer's Elbow.
Lateral Epicondylitis	Inflammation of the wrist extensors at the lateral epicondyle (outside of the elbow). Caused by an overload to the wrist extensors. In pole, this injury is often caused in the lower hand of a full bracket hold when the athlete is either already injured or relatively weak or inflexible in the wrist and finger extensors. Under these circumstances, pain is usually first noticed in the middle of the lateral forearm and later travels to the elbow. Also known as Tennis Elbow.
Abdominal Muscle Strain	Injury of abdominal muscle. Without adequate stretching and balanced development, abdominal muscles can become tight on the opposite side of the dominant arm or leg, increasing likelihood of strain
Intercostal Strain	Strain of the muscles located between ribs. Can be caused by an imbalance in core strength.
Costovertebral Joint Sprain	Dislocation and/or damage to the cartilage and/or connective tissue surrounding the costovertebral joint (joint where a rib meets the backbone). Pain is usually felt on one side of the spine, back, and/or rib cage.
DeQuervain's Syndrome and ECU Tendonitis	Inflammation of tendons in the wrist caused by repetitive twisting, backward flexion, and gripping.

Musculoskeletal injury is of particular significance to pole athletes. Kibler and Chandler state that "microscopic muscle damage occurs with intense muscle contractions or with tensile overload to the muscle and tendon unit...eccentric exercise has been shown to produce considerably more damage to skeletal muscle than other types of exercise (19)." These types of intense, high load, eccentric contractions are the hallmark of advanced Pole fitness. With this in mind, pole athletes and instructors should take special care to avoid injury.

- **Impact on self-efficacy and emotional health**

As with physical responses to stress, there is also a large amount of variability in the degree that stress (training and psychosocial) affects the emotional status of different individuals. There are, however, several frequent and widespread psychological consequences of overtraining.

Table 4.4: Possible Emotional Consequences of Overtraining
• Feelings of Depression
• General Apathy
• Decreased self-esteem
• Emotional instability
• Difficulty concentrating
• Sensitivity to stress
• Changes in personality
• Anxiety
• Irritability
• Increased feelings of frustration and disappointment

Morgan et al. demonstrated this in a summary of studies over a 10 year period during which research was conducted at the University of Wisconsin by administering the Profile of Moods States (POMS) to 400 swimmers and other collegiate athletes along with non-athletes. Through analysis of training and POMS data, the researchers identified several patterns of mood disturbance with training. One conclusion they came to was that "stale [or over-trained] athletes, defined by mood and performance deterioration, demonstrate symptoms similar to those seen in clinical depression (27, 30)."

In another study by Fry et al., a negative impact on self-efficacy was seen after the implementation of a two week, high intensity training program. Although the training difficulty of the program did not increase throughout the two week period, "perceptions of anticipated lifting success were significantly decreased by day 8 (8,10)." In other words, as overtraining was induced, the athletes began to lose confidence in themselves and their abilities, even though the actual difficulty levels were not increased.

It's also important to note that elite athletes are not immune to the psychological consequences of overtraining. Through the use of the POMS, Meyers and Whelan evaluated the emotional changes in elite adolescent and young adult weightlifters over a 1 week period of intense training. By the end of the week, mood and psychological well-being had noticeably deteriorated as the athletes neared a state of overtraining (27).

It is actually no wonder that overtraining can result in mood deterioration and depressive like symptoms. If you've ever experienced pregnancy or pre-menstrual syndrome, or been around someone who has, you know firsthand that hormones affect the way we feel emotionally. Exercise induces complicated interactions between the endocrine system (hormone system) and the rest of the body. Depending on the characteristics of the training bout, hormone levels in the blood are elevated or reduced as part of the body's effort to protect itself, deal with the immediate stress, and adapt for future applications of stress. To a certain point, many of these hormones have a positive effect on mood.

Opioid peptides ("feel good" endorphins), for example, are increased in the blood during exercise. Growth Hormone, Thyroid and parathyroid hormones, sex hormones, and glucocorticoids (Cortisol) levels are also increased in the blood during normal exercise bouts, producing physical and emotional boosts (7). The problem, however, comes when an athlete enters into a state of overtraining. In this state, complicated hormone interaction becomes altered and can no longer provide its typical services as the body strays farther and farther away from homeostasis. For example, Keizer states that "very demanding exercise may depress the nocturnal Growth Hormone secretion, which then resembles the pattern observed in obese subjects, depressive patients, and in the elderly (17)."

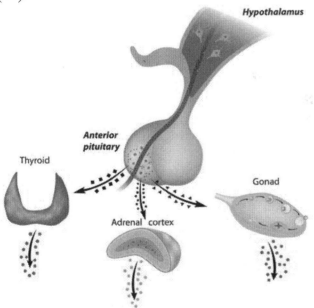

Another important hormonal system affected by too much stress is the Hypothalamic-Pituitary-Adrenal (HPA) axis. The release of CRH neurons (specific chemicals within the brain) is governed by the HPA axis and is increased as stress is applied to the body. Unfortunately for those who push themselves too hard, CRH has profound effects on mood, from arousal and fear to anxiety and depression (17). Reasonable exercise can definitely have a positive effect on psychological health but training too much can lead to a devastating state of emotional deterioration.

- **Additional hormonal/endocrine system effects**

The lack of hormonal homeostasis in the body due to overtraining can also have harmful physical and performance effects. Growth Hormone (GH) secretion, for example, is suppressed by high levels of corticoids (stress induced hormones). Since Growth Hormone stimulates protein synthesis (i.e. muscle and tissue building), a decrease in GH levels will result in increased fatigue and longer recovery times post training (5,7,17).

Hormones that are ultimately controlled by different parts of the brain (i.e. Hypothalamus and Pituitary gland) can also negatively affect the overtrained athlete. Increased production of glucocorticoids (along with a decrease in testosterone levels) caused by a stress/recovery imbalance creates a catabolic environment in the body. This environment leads to protein degradation (muscle wasting). It is obvious that, without adequate recovery, this effect would increase fatigue and decrease strength and performance over time.

Table 4.5: Additional Hormonal Driven Effects of Overtraining
• Protein degradation/muscle catabolism
• Decreased protein synthesis
• Sleep disturbance
• Increased resting heart rate
• Changes in metabolism
• Amenorrhea (loss of menstrual period)
• Decrease in exercise recovery rate
• Decrease in sex drive

Interestingly, exercise induced changes in hormone levels and secretions do not necessarily go back to normal after the training bout is finished. If the body is consistently not allowed enough time to recover before additional training stresses are applied, it will be in a constant state of imbalance. The endocrine system will be working overtime to try and attain a level of homeostasis. The greater the state of imbalance within the body, the more extreme and abnormal the endocrine system reacts in order to keep the body from completely shutting down. Nocturnal hormonal secretions are even affected, which helps explain why many overtrained athletes have trouble sleeping (17,18).

Preventing Overtraining

The fundamental theory behind preventing overtraining is simple: incorporate sufficient recovery time and variability before applying additional training stress. If overtraining symptoms do start to develop, these should be immediately addressed with additional rest and recovery tactics. The trick is to know exactly what this means for the individual athlete in varying training circumstances. Unfortunately, sufficient recovery time can vary tremendously between athletes and different training routines. Specific overtraining symptoms also differ vastly. In order for the individual athlete to prevent overtraining and maintain an optimum stress recovery balance, they must pay close attention to their own psychological and physiological state in association with their performance and level of applied training stress. Preventing overtraining requires the athlete to honestly look at how they feel, how they are performing, and how much they are training. Once the first signs of too much stress or not enough recovery are experienced, the athlete must pull back on training or overtraining will develop.

It can be extremely tempting to push too hard in pole where performance gains are seen quickly and new, exciting tricks are just within reach. Unfortunately, as Rountree mentions in her book on athletic recovery, "overtraining is reversible only by a prolonged period of rest, one that can last for weeks or even months. Hence your athletic success depends on purposely avoiding pushing yourself into such a state (38)."

Table 4.6: Signs That May Indicate the Onset of Overtraining
• Persistent performance stagnation or decrease
• Feelings of pain or soreness in the tendons or joints
• Unbalanced soreness in muscles
• Persistent fatigue
• Lack of motivation or discouragement in training
• Pulled muscles
• Elevated resting heart rate
• Increased irritability
• Depressed mood
• Sleep disturbances

One common reason for avoiding extra rest is the fear that breaking from training will result in a loss of previous performance gains. While it is true that gains in aerobic endurance are lost fairly quickly when training is ceased, this is generally not the case with strength and anaerobic endurance gains. In fact, as stated by Foss et al, "it is generally agreed that strength and [anaerobic] endurance once developed, subside at slower rates than they were developed (7)." The amount of strength retention during time off from training is actually quite impressive and supported by numerous studies (3,26,28,35,36). One of these studies, for example, showed that strength gains from a 3 day per week, 3 week long strength training program were still present after 6 weeks of rest following the training program (3,7). Eventually strength gains will decline with the lack of training stimulus, but not nearly as quickly as one might think. Don't let the fear of losing progress prevent you from getting the rest and recovery your body needs. It's better to invest the relatively short amount of time in recovery at the first signs of overtraining than to train through them and end up out of the game for weeks or months.

If you do find yourself caught in a perpetuation of overtraining, or develop a serious injury, don't panic. Unless the body has been severely damaged beyond repair, with appropriate rest, it will heal itself and eventually come back into a state of homeostasis. Depending on the degree of overtraining and injury state, this can take a substantial amount of time. Unfortunately, the overtrained athlete doesn't have any other choice. Continued training will only advance athletic deterioration. The time, however long it is, dedicated toward allowing the body to recover and heal will always be more beneficial to an athlete and their performance in the long run.

Table 4.7: Suggestions to Prevent Overtraining
• Set appropriate goals
• Prepare non-exercise activities to deal with anxiety or boredom
• Recognize the difference between soreness and injury
• Take a break from training when you feel something is amiss in your training or body
• Account for physical and psychological stress during activities of daily life
• Rest on rest days
• Track mood, sleep quality, fatigue, and performance levels
• Be honest with yourself and rest when you even suspect you need to!
• Have patience with yourself and faith in the process of improved performance through recovery
• Include additional time off each month in addition to rest days during the week
• Attempt to reduce non-training psychosocial stress as much as possible
• Use imagery as a substitute for physical training when extra rest is warranted

Continuing Education Questions

1. Why are pole athletes susceptible to overtraining? How does a typical strength training program compare to pole?
2. What are some of the factors that lead to overtraining?
3. Why is it not a good idea to mimic the training plan of an elite athlete?
4. What are some of the culturally driven factors that can lead to overtraining?
5. What happens when the body doesn't have enough glucose/glycogen to fuel glycolysis?
6. What is muscle catabolism/wasting and what effects does it have on athletic performance?
7. How does taking nonsteroidal anti-inflammatory drugs too often affect athletic development and performance?
8. What are some of the common outcomes of overtraining?
9. Why is a state of accumulated fatigue a dangerous place for an athlete to be?
10. What are some of the common overtraining injuries seen in pole?
11. Why is it critical to return to training gradually after experiencing an injury?
12. What is the fundamental theory behind preventing overtraining?
13. Is it true that strength is lost very quickly during times of inactivity?

References and Additional Sources

1. Anderson, M. K., Martin, M., & Hall, S. J. (1995). Sports injury management. Baltimore, MD: Williams & Wilkins.
2. Barnett, A. (2006). Using Recovery Modalities between Training Sessions in Elite Athletes. Sports Medicine, 36(9), 781-796. doi: 10.2165/00007256-200636090-00005

3. Berger, R. A. (1965). Comparison of the effect of various weight training loads. Research Quarterly for Exercise and Sport, (36), 141-146.

4. Berning, J. R. (1998). Energy Intake, Diet, and Muscle Wasting. In R. B. Kreider, A. C. Fry, & M. L. O'Toole (Eds.), Overtraining in sport (pp. 275-288). Champaign, IL: Human Kinetics.

5. Bompa, T. O., & Haff, C. G. (2009). Periodization: Theory and methodology of training (5th ed.). Champaign, IL: Human Kinetics.

6. Calais-Germain, B., & Anderson, S. (1993). Anatomy of movement. Seattle, WA: Eastland Press.

7. Foss, M. L., & Keteyian, S. J. (1998). Fox's physiological basis for exercise and sport. (6th ed.). Boston, MA: WCB/McGraw-Hill.

8. Fry, A. C. (1998). The role of training intensity in resistance exercise overtraining and overreaching. In R. B. Kreider, A. C. Fry, & M. L. O'Toole (Eds.), Overtraining in sport (pp. 107-127). Champaign, IL: Human Kinetics.

9. Fry, A. C., Kraemer, W. J., Van Borselen, F., Lynch, J. M., Marsit, J. L., Roy, E. P., Knuttgen, H. G. (1994). Performance decrements with high-intensity resistance exercise overtraining. Medicine and Science in Sports and Exercise, (26), 1165-1173.

10. Fry, M. D., Fry, A. C., & Kraemer, W. J. (1996). Self-efficacy responses to short-term high intensity resistance exercise overtraining. Lecture presented at International Conference on Overtraining in Sport: Physiological, Psychological, and Biomedical Considerations, Memphis. In Overtraining in sport. (1998). Champaign, IL: Human Kinetics.

11. Gould, D., Greenleaf, C., Chung, Y., & Guinan, D. (2002). A survey of U.S. Atlanta and Nangano Olympians: Variables perceived to influence performance. Research Quarterly for

Exercise and Sport, (73), 175-186.

12. Gulick, D. T., Kimura, I. F., Sitler, M., Paolone, A., & Kelly, J. D. (1996). Various treatment techniques on signs and symptoms of delayed onset muscle soreness. Journal of Athletic Training, (31), 145-152.

13. Guten, G. N. (2005). Injuries in outdoor recreation: Understanding, prevention, and treatment. Guilford, CT: FalconGuide.

14. Hatfield, B. D., & Brody, E. B. (1994). The psychology of athletic preparation and performance: The mental management of physical resources. In T. R. Baechle (Ed.), Essentials of strength training and conditioning (pp. 163-185). Champaign, IL: Human Kinetics.

15. Hodges, N. J., Hayes, S., Horn, R. R., & Williams, A. M. (2005). Changes in coordination, control and outcome as a result of extended practice on a novel motor skill. Ergonomics, (48), 1672-1685.

16. Hooper, S. L., & Mackinnon, L. T. (1995). Monitoring Overtraining in Athletes. Sports Medicine, 20(5), 321-327. doi: 10.2165/00007256-199520050-00003

17. Keizer, H. A. (1998). Neuroendocrine aspects of overtraining. In R. B. Kreider, A. C. Fry, & M. L. O'Toole (Eds.), Overtraining in sport (pp. 145-159). Champaign, IL: Human Kinetics.

18. Kern, W. B., Perras, B., Wodick, R., Fehm, H. L., & Born, J. (1995). Hormonal secretion during nighttime sleep indicating stress of daytime exercise. Journal of Applied Physiology, (79), 1461-1468.

19. Kibler, W. B., & Chandler, T. J. (1998). Musculoskeletal and orthopedic considerations. In R. B. Kreider, A. C. Fry, & M. L. O'Toole (Eds.), Overtraining in sport (pp. 169-190). Champaign, IL: Human Kinetics.

20. Kraemer, W. J., & Nindl, B. C. (1998). Factors involved with

overtraining for strength and power. In R. B. Kreider, A. C. Fry, & M. L. O'Toole (Eds.), Overtraining in sport (pp. 69-86). Champaign, IL: Human Kinetics.

21. Kraemer, W. J. (1994). Neuroendocrine responses to resistance exercise. In T. R. Baechle (Ed.), Essentials of strength training and conditioning (pp. 86-103). Champaign, IL: Human Kinetics.

22. Kreider, R. B. (1998). Central fatigue hypothesis and overtraining. In R. B. Kreider, A. C. Fry, & M. L. O'Toole (Eds.), Overtraining in sport (pp. 309-331). Champaign, IL: Human Kinetics.

23. Kreider, R. B., Fry, A. C., & O'Toole, M. L. (Eds.). (1998). Overtraining in sport. Champaign, IL: Human Kinetics.

24. Leiber, R. L., & Friden, J. (1993). Muscle damage is not a function of muscle force but active muscle strain. Journal of Applied Physiology, (74), 520-526.

25. Marieb, E. N., & Hoehn, K. (2010). Human anatomy and physiology (8th ed., pp. 911-954). Glenview, IL: Pearson/ Benjamin Cummings.

26. McMorris, R., & Elkins, E. (1954). A study of production and evaluation of muscular hypertrophy. Archives of Physical Medicine and Rehabilitation, (35), 420-426.

27. Meyers, A. W., & Whelan, J. P. (1998). A systemic model for understanding psychosocial influences in overtraining. In R. B. Kreider, A. C. Fry, & M. L. O'Toole (Eds.), Overtraining in sport (pp. 335-364). Champaign, IL: Human Kinetics.

28. Morehouse, C. (1967). Development and maintenance of isometric strength of subjects with diverse initial strengths. Research Quarterly for Exercise and Sport, (38), 449-456.

29. Morgan, W., O'Connor, P., Sparling, P., & Pate, R. (1987). Psychological Characterization of the Elite Female Distance Runners*. International Journal of Sports Medicine, 08(S 2), S124-S131. doi: 10.1055/s-2008-1025717

30. Morgan, W. P., Brown, D. R., Raglin, J. S., O'Connor, P. J., & Ellickson, K. A. (1987). Psychological monitoring of over-training and staleness. British Journal of Sports Medicine, 21 (3), 107-114. doi: 10.1136/bjsm.21.3.107

31. Morgan, W. P., O'Connor, P. J., Ellickson, K. A., & Bradley, P. W. (1988). Personality structure, mood states, and perfor-mance in elite male distance runners. International Journal of Sport Psychology, (19), 247-263.

32. O'Toole, M. L. (1998). Overreaching and overtraining in en-durance athletes. In R. B. Kreider, A. C. Fry, & M. L. O'Toole (Eds.), Overtraining in sport (p. 11). Champaign, IL: Human Kinetics.

33. Pecina, M., & Bojanic, I. (1993). Overuse injuries of the mus-culoskeletal system. Boca Raton, FL: CRC Press.

34. Raglin, J. S., Sawamura, S., Alexiou, S., Hassmen, P., & Kentta, G. (2000). Training practices in 13-18-year-old swim-mers: A cross-cultural study. Pediatric Exercise Science, (12), 61-70.

35. Rasch, P., & Morehouse, L. (1957). Effect of static and dy-namic exercises on muscular strength and hypertrophy. Jour-nal of Applied Physiology, (11), 29-34.

36. Rasch, P. (1971). Isometric exercise and gains of muscle strength. In R. J. Shephard (Ed.), Frontiers of fitness. Spring-field, IL: Thomas.

37. Richardson, S. O., Andersen, M. B., & Morris, T. (2008). Overtraining athletes: Personal journeys in sport. Champaign, IL: Human Kinetics.

38. Rountree, S. H. (2011). The athlete's guide to recovery: Rest, relax, and restore for peak performance. Boulder, CO: Ve-loPress.

39. Rowbottom, D. G., Keast, D., & Morton, A. R. (1998). Moni-toring and preventing of overreaching and overtraining in en-durance athletes. In R. B. Kreider, A. C. Fry, & M. L. O'Toole

(Eds.), Overtraining in sport (pp. 107-123). Champaign, IL: Human Kinetics.

40. Sherman, W. M., Jacobs, K. A., & Leenders, N. (1998). Carbohydrate metabolism during endurance exercise. In R. B. Kreider, A. C. Fry, & M. L. O'Toole (Eds.), Overtraining in sport (pp. 289-307). Champaign, IL: Human Kinetics.

41. Soltow, Q. A., Betters, J. L., Sellman, J. E., Lira, V. A., Long, J. D., & Criswell, D. S. (2006). Ibuprofen Inhibits Skeletal Muscle Hypertrophy in Rats. Medicine & Science in Sports & Exercise, 38(5), 840-846. doi: 10.1249/01.mss.0000218142.98704.66

42. Stone, M. H., & Conley, M. S. (1994). Bioenergetics. In T. R. Baechle (Ed.), Essentials of strength training and conditioning (pp. 67-81). Champaign, IL: Human Kinetics.

43. Stone, M. H., & Fry, A. C. (1998). Increased training volume in strength/power athletes. In R. B. Kreider, A. C. Fry, & M. L. O'Toole (Eds.), Overtraining in sport (pp. 96-102). Champaign, IL: Human Kinetics.

44. Stone, M. H. (1994). Eating disorders. In T. R. Baechle (Ed.), Essentials of strength training and conditioning (pp. 238-242). Champaign, IL: Human Kinetics.

45. Stone, M. H. (1994). Nutritional factors in performance and health. In T. R. Baechle (Ed.), Essentials of strength training and conditioning (pp. 210-226). Champaign, IL: Human Kinetics.

46. Stone, M., Keith, R., Kearney, J., Fleck, S., Wilson, G., & Triplett, N. (1991). Overtraining: A review of the signs, symptoms and possible causes. The Journal of Strength and Conditioning Research, 5(1), 35-50. doi: 10.1519/1533-4287(1991)0052.3.CO;2

47. Trappe, T. A., White, F., Lambert, C. P., Cesar, D., Hellerstein, M., & Evans, W. J. (2002). Effect of ibuprofen and acetaminophen on post exercise muscle protein synthesis.

American Journal of Physiology-Endocrinology and Metabolism, (282), E551-E556.

Chapter 5
Training Program Design

Purpose/Goals

As has been mentioned, there are numerous exercise programs available that prescribe very specific movements, volumes, and intensities to be performed consistently to obtain the "rock hard abbs" or "Buns of Steel." These types of programs are popular sellers because they tell a person exactly what to do to get the advertised results. Unfortunately, as we've seen, training and the way it affects the body is complicated and individual. A "one size fits all" training program will not produce the same results for everyone, and unfortunately, most often leads to burnout, staleness and/or overtraining. Many are lured into popular exercise prescriptions because, beyond a good looking body, they aren't sure what they want. If they do have specific performance goals, they may not know how to train to achieve them. Following a popular exercise program can make people "feel" like they are doing something to "get fit." The real question here, though, is what does "get fit" mean and what is "getting fit" going to do for me?

In order to attain real athletic performance goals, the athlete must first know what those goals are. Without a purpose, athletic training is meaningless. As Bompa states, "The intent of training is to increase the athlete's skills and work capacity to optimize athletic performance (4)." If there are no athletic performance goals, then there is no point in training. Further, different athletic goals require different types of training. An individual who aspires to maintain a base level of fitness and health benefits will train much differently than an athlete preparing for a national pole competition, who will also train much differently from a triathlete, or marathon runner. Even further, each athlete or aspiring athlete is completely unique. Their specific physiology, athletic abilities, training history, and life stressors will affect the way they respond to a training program. In order for an athlete to attain their own personal best, their training program must be unique to them and their goals (3,4,13,16).

With all this in mind, the first step to designing a training program is to establish goals. These don't have to be overly specific or complicated. The point is to create a purpose or objective that will guide the type of training activities and 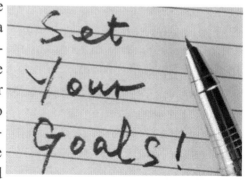 decisions that make up a program. The following are some questions that can be considered when constructing a goal for training.

- Do I want to participate in multiple sports or just pole?
- Do I want to compete in pole?
- Do I want to compete in other sports?
- What is my current athletic level?
- Do I have any previous injuries that may affect how I train
- Are there any specific competitions that I would like to enter
- What is my desired time frame for changes in performance ability?
- Do I want to teach pole?
- What level of athleticism do I want to attain?
- Do I want to become an advanced, elite pole athlete or am I fine with just poling from time to time for fun?
- Do I have access to instruction and/or coaching?

Depending on the answers to these questions, goals for training can be developed and used to design a training program. Some examples of possible goals are listed below.

- Participate weekly in pole and other various activities as a means to maintain general fitness and camaraderie with others.
- Gain enough stamina and skill to periodically perform intermediate to advanced tricks for friends and family.
- Become proficient at beginning and intermediate pole moves by the end of the year.
- Obtain an elite level of stamina, strength, and skill to perform or teach at an advanced level.

As time goes on, goals can be revised or completely changed. Keeping up to date goals will not only ensure that a training program is in line with these goals, but will also provide direction and purpose in training and in life.

Periodization

As has been discussed several times, beneficial training requires alternating periods of stress and recovery. In addition, monotonous training (i.e. training the same way all the time) and continuous stress increases (linear loading) must also be avoided in order to obtain optimal performance levels. The concept of Periodization, as presented by Bompa et al., is a great way to create a framework for an effective training program (3,4,21,25). Periodization ensures that a training program is adequately varied and provides stress/recovery balance.

Periodization consists of several specific training cycles nested within each other. Bompa (3,4) suggests that athletes begin planning their program with an annual plan. The simplest of these, the monocycle, breaks a year into three different phases of training: preparatory, competitive, and a transition phase. During the preparatory phase, the athlete focuses on building overall strength, endurance, and flexibility. After the preparatory phase, the athlete can adjust their training to focus more on skills, technique, and increased intensity to enhance athletic ability and/or to prepare for competition. Once through this phase, the annual cycle is completed with a transition phase during which the athlete focuses on rest and recovery to compensate for the intense competitive phase and to prepare for a new preparatory phase in the next year.

To guide training within the three phases of the annual monocycle, Bompa (3,4) describes a shorter cycle called a macrocycle which lasts two to seven weeks. Each macrocycle can be designed to help focus training efforts on the specific phase of the annual cycle that the athlete is in (i.e. preparatory, competitive, or transition). Within a macrocycle is the microcycle, the weekly (or three to seven days) training breakdown that is guided by the objectives of the macrocycle (which is guided by the objectives of the differ

Table 5.1: Periodized Annual Training Program

Phase of Monocycle (3 separate training focuses over one year)	Macrocycles (2-7 week periods of varied volume and intensity)	Microcycles (1 week periods providing specific training direction for the macrocycles and annual plan. The Microcyles are made up of individual workouts.)
Transition Phase	Recovery	Flexibility
		Off
	Medium	Active Rest
		Multilateral
Competitive Phase	Recovery	Off/Peak
		Active Rest
	Hard	Power
		Power
	Hard	Endurance
		Strength
Preparatory Phase	Recovery	Off
		Active Rest
	Hard	Endurance
		Strength
	Medium	Multilateral
		Multilateral

ent phases of the annual plan). Within the microcycle are the individual workouts which should also be designed for the particular training phase in focus.

Designing a program with Periodization concepts can become as detailed and complicated as you want, but complex planning and details are really not necessary or overly beneficial for the large majority of athletes. All most athletes need is to have a basic periodized structure in their minds to help guide decisions on training volumes, intensity, technical practice, and rest. Throughout the year, there should be a time when the athlete focuses on building base levels of fitness, strength, and endurance (Preparatory phase of the annual plan), a time when intensity is increased and focus shifts toward technique and competitive development (competitive phase), and a time when training is focused on restoration and preparation for the next year (transition phase). Every few weeks (macrocycle) the athlete should switch things up a bit. Taking a week off after three or four is good way to do this. The specific workouts conducted throughout the week (microcycle) should be designed to support the specific focus of the macrocycle and the particular time of year.

Intuition and Body Awareness

As tempting as it is to prescribe "the" periodized workout plan for pole athletes, there are just too many variables in individual goals, physiology, athletic history and condition, etc. to solely rely on a generic periodized plan. As has been discussed, each individual will react uniquely to a given training program. The same stimulus applied to athletes with similar athletic abilities and multilateral development can cause one athlete to obtain optimal performance but overtrain another (4,16,23). In addition, different individual goals necessitate varied training program design. A person striving for an international title must train differently than someone who is training for different types of sports or is only seeking a general multilateral fitness base.

With so much variability from person to person, how then can an athlete or aspiring athlete train to achieve their greatest performance potential? To answer this question we must simply return to the basic principle of training: the body adapts based on the stresses that it experiences. For optimum performance enhancement, the athlete must experience the perfect balance of stress and recovery for their body. No generic program can provide this for an individual because only the individual can truly know where their body is in the stress/recovery balance. Fortunately, with practice, an athlete can become intimately aware of exactly where they are on the stress/recovery continuum. They can use this awareness within a periodized framework to apply varying degrees and types of stress or recovery at the moment that will benefit their body's performance the most.

Contrary to many of the popular messages and images, using intuition and body awareness to guide training is not an athletic copout. An athlete in tune with their body will be able to tell when they need to rest. By recognizing their position on the training adaptation curve and acting on it, they will be setting themselves up for optimum adaptation and performance enhancement. If, on the other hand, the athlete ignores their intuition and body sensation because they think they "should" train harder, they will stress their body beyond the optimal balance of stress and recovery, resulting in prolonged recovery times, fatigue, decreases in performance, and injury. Ignoring or blocking out body intuition and sensation is where overtraining and the consequent decreases in performance originate. Intuition and body awareness take into account all of the many factors that can affect an athlete's ability to train and recover. This not only simplifies the whole process of program design, but allows each athlete to achieve his or her personal best.

Intuitive training can seem a bit more ambiguous than always completing a straight forward program with a predetermined number of exercises, sets, and repetitions but this does not mean that it is not based on a solid scientific foundation. As we've begun to see, the human body is incredibly intricate and complicated and its full examination is beyond the scope of this book. There are, however, a few physiological sources discussed below to support the validity of using intuition and body awareness to guide athletic training.

Without measuring a workout based on external indicators (i.e. time, reps, sets), one of the most obvious indicators that the body needs rest is the presence of fatigue. We know intuitively that when we exercise we eventually begin to feel worn out, but why does this happen? One physiological explanation is the central fatigue theory (15,17,19,20). During prolonged exercise, skeletal muscle begins to take amino acids (proteins including glutamine and the BCAAs leucine, isoleucine, and valine) from the blood in order to maintain the energy supply that is being demanded by the muscles. At the same time, free tryptophan (an essential amino acid) levels in the blood are increased. BCAAs and free tryptophan tend to compete for entry into the brain, so a decrease in BCAA levels along with an increase in tryptophan during exercise results in an increase in tryptophan levels in the brain. Once inside the brain, tryptophan promotes the formation of the neurotransmitter 5-hydroxytryptamine (5-HT) which then, depending on concentrations and conditions in the brain, induces tiredness, psychological perception of fatigue, and reduction in muscle power output. As exercise continues, more BCAAs are removed from the blood, increasing the fatigue effects of tryptophan in the brain.

In other words, an athlete in tune with their body can determine the optimum amount of training stress to apply based on the accumulating fatigue they experience in their body. This fascinating link between physiological reactions to exercise within the body and psychological perceptions and intuitive sensations of fatigue provides fantastic substantiation to the practice of using intuition and body awareness to guide training.

Another link between physiology and body awareness is found in joint and muscle sensation (5,8). The body is full of millions of nerves and proprioceptors. These receptors recognize different conditions experienced throughout the body and send messages to the central nervous system (the spinal cord and brain) to convey what is happening. We experience this reaction as sensation or feeling in our body. When a muscle is pulled or torn, for example, nerves within the muscle send a "pain" message to the central nervous system which results in the feeling of pain in the injured muscle. The action of nerves and proprioceptors provide the physiological basis for body sensations such as pain, discomfort, pressure, and balance. The key to using these sensations in intuitive exercise or training, is to know what each of the experienced

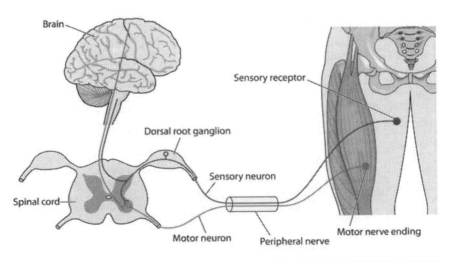

sensations mean to your individual body. Especially in pole fitness, some level of pain and discomfort is expected and even necessary in training. Unfortunately, too much pain and discomfort is indicative of overtraining and can lead to serious injury, loss of training time, and decreased performance. Apart from injury and obvious signs of fatigue or pain, only the individual athlete will know how much is too much. The ability to determine this comes as the athlete makes a conscious effort to recognize the different sensations they feel and the outcomes those sensations seem to correlate with. It may be necessary to experiment by mentally (or physically) logging varying training volumes and intensities along with the physiological and psychological outcomes experienced in order to become intimately aware of the sensations experienced during the most beneficial application of training stress and recovery. Below is a list contrasting sensations felt with typical soreness from training versus injurious pain. Additional guides for training intuition and sensation are provided at the end of this chapter.

Table 5.2: Soreness vs. Injurous Pain	
Soreness	Injurious pain
• Tenderness in the center or throughout major muscle groups • May peak 1-2 days after training but fades quickly after 3 days • Soreness felt evenly on both sides of the body	• Pain localized toward a joint • Sharp pain • Pain that develops immediately during training • Nagging pain that doesn't seem to go away over time • Pain that is exacerbated by specific movement or exercise

A final interesting physiological source related to intuitive exercise is involuntary inhibition. There are several mechanisms in the body that automatically react and activate sensations to protect us from injury and other consequences of overtraining

(2,5,8). A great example of these is Golgi tendon organs (GTOs) and muscle spindles. As discussed earlier, these proprioceptors act in conjunction with one another to ensure that a muscle isn't stretched too far. When a muscle is stretched, whether during active stretching or an exercise activity, the muscle spindles react by conveying a sensation of pain and at the same time inducing a contraction in the muscle to prevent it from being pulled further or torn. When a muscle experiences a sufficient amount of stretch, the GTOs are also activated, resulting in muscle relaxation or contraction inhibition. As stated by Foss et al., "this can be interpreted as a protective function in that during attempts to lift extremely heavy loads that could cause injury, the tendon organs cause a relaxation of the muscles (8)." When an athlete feels the sensations of muscle spindles and Golgi tendon organs they can act accordingly to prevent injury. An athlete can also use awareness of the occurrence of contraction inhibition (i.e. the muscles not doing what is expected or desired) to monitor, evaluate, and modify training volume and intensity (6,9,10,22).

Before getting too wrapped up in worrying about how to perfect your knowledge and application of the myriad of training related sensations and physiological reactions and experiences, take a quick look at a young child exercising. Before they've been inundated with social norms and expectations, stresses of life, and inaccurate, inauspicious ideas about exercise and training, children perfectly embody the unadulterated concept of intuitive exercise. They move when and how then want. They do what feels good and stop what doesn't. They sit and they squirm, they run around, climb on things, and hop up and down. Then, when they don't "feel" like "exercising" any more, they stop. No one has to tell them how much to run or how many rungs on the jungle gym to climb, they just know. These children are some of the fittest people around. If we can scrape away all of the jargon we've been inundated with and access the intuition of a young child, we will also be able to access the superior, injury free fitness level that a young child experiences.

Role of Self-Belief and the Power of the Mind

A final important component of an effective individualized training program is a healthy degree of self-efficacy and a positive attitude. As stated by Bompa et al., "psychological factors, such as self-confidence, morale, desire, and beliefs, appear to be significantly related to the athlete's ability to perform or develop skills (4)." This makes sense when we remember that physiological and psychological stresses are cumulative. High levels of psychological stress combined with athletic training can create an imbalance in the athlete's stress/recovery balance (4,18). If prolonged, this will result in fatigue and performance stagnation or decrements. Damaging amounts of psychological stress develop when an athlete holds critical, negative self-beliefs. Low confidence, self-rejection, unrealistic expectations, self-berating, and conditional self-love all demand athletic perfection. This unrealistic expectation is stressful enough by itself, but when perfection is inevitably not reached, a crushing cycle is closed as the athlete reinforces negative self-beliefs.

An optimal response to a training program occurs when an athlete can manage training and psychosocial stresses with wholesome self-worth, positive and realistic beliefs and expectations, and an encouraging and confident inner voice. These not only decrease the amount of psychological stress experienced during the training experience, but prevent a backlash of unproductive reactions when performance inevitably isn't at its peak. If you want to be great, don't beat yourself up for not being perfect. No athlete is perfect. We are each on our own continuum of development.

Specific Training Suggestions for Pole Athletes

Recreational poler:

How an athlete trains once again largely depends on their goals. For the casual pole participant who doesn't have aspirations to progress beyond beginner level technique, a concentrated effort on training program development is not necessary. The activities consistent with these goals include floor work, dance, transitions, and beginner spins, practiced one to two times a week in a non-competitive, leisurely environment. This activity will help establish a healthy, respectable level of multilateral development which will enable the participant to advance enough to enjoy smooth and consistent beginner level pole and dance. Because this level of participation generally involves less potential for stress overload and is less concerned with performance enhancement, even a person new to the idea of intuitive exercise can rely on body sensations and awareness to guide their activity levels. This, in fact, will be great practice in the event that more advanced goals are developed.

Pole athlete with advanced performance goals:

As goals become more focused on attaining an advanced level of skill and fitness, training practices will necessitate more careful consideration and implementation. If applied incorrectly, training with an emphasis on increasing performance can lead to counterproductive symptoms of overtraining including injury, fatigue, and performance decline. Training solely based on intuition is still very much possible at this level of training and really is the ultimate goal. An athlete who is intimately aware of the relationships between their training practices and their body's reaction experienced through sensations and intuitions is able to perfectly individualize their training program. No time is wasted in extra recovery from doing too much nor is there a performance involution (decrease) from not training enough. By listening to their body, an intuitive athlete can tell when and how much to push and rest in order to maintain the optimal balance of stress and recovery for their body.

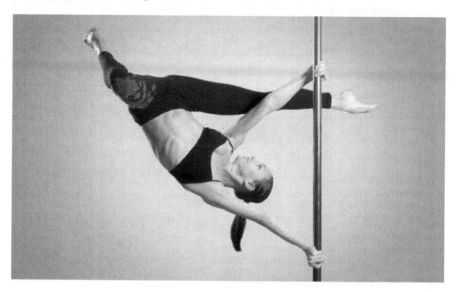

For many athletes who aren't yet experts at using body cues to guide training decisions, it can be helpful to have some sort of framework or guidance to keep them on the right track. As an athlete trains within an appropriate framework, they will become more aware of the most optimal way for their body to train. They will begin to see what feels and works best for their development.

- **Multilateral Development**

The first step in any training program is to ensure that an adequate level of multilateral development is established (3,4). This base level of fitness consists of balanced strength, flexibility, endurance, and agility and serves as a foundation for specific athletic development. Without this foundation, athletes are hugely susceptible to injury and are much less likely to reach their performance potential (4). In pole, continued multilateral development can be acquired through a thorough progression of each pole skill level. Even with an athlete who is starting pole with an elevated fitness level, time should be spent training in lower skill levels until enough balance, strength, flexibility, and endurance have been obtained to execute these skills with control on both dominant and non-dominant sides of the body. It is especially tempting in pole to accelerate the development of specific skills while neglecting others. Once an athlete is able to execute an advanced trick on their dominant side, it is tempting to continue advancing in trick progression on that same side without training the other side of the body. As new advanced tricks come into the realm of possibility, it's challenging to go back and work on the other side, but balanced strength development will, in the long run, prevent injury, enhance athletic performance, and result in well-rounded technical mastery.

- **Methodology and Volume**

In a serious athletic training program, the concept of specificity of training should direct what the athlete does to train. For pole this means that training should largely focus on the anaerobic metabolic system, flexibility, and high-intensity endurance. Because of the concept of specificity of training, the best way to train for a specific skill or sport is to practice that specific skill or sport. Weight training, for example, does address the specific bioenergetic pathways that are also seen in pole and can improve strength and endurance, but it does not necessarily create the same physiological adaptations that training on the pole does. Programs containing a majority of non-pole type training can be created to effectively produce positive results in pole performance, but if the ultimate goal is to increase pole performance, training on the pole is the most efficient way to build applicable strength, endurance, skill, and technique. Moderate weight training in addition to pole can be a good way of maintaining multilateral development and physiological balance but is not essential to meet enhanced performance goals in pole.

A common mistake in training for pole is including excessive levels of aerobic training. As mentioned previously, the body adapts based on the specific types of stresses that it experiences. If an athlete sufficiently trains their aerobic energy system, the body will adapt by enhancing the efficiency and predominance of the aerobic system. Unfortunately, this comes at the expense of the performance of the anaerobic system. Since pole is largely dominated by high intensity anaerobic activity, adding consistent aerobic training such as jogging is likely to stagnate or decrease performance in pole (4,7,8,12,14).

In an effort to gain strength, pole athletes may also be tempted to include excessive amounts of callisthenic training (i.e. sit-ups, push-ups, crunches, etc.) in their training programs. These exercises are good for warming up the body and for multilateral development in moderation, but excessive application in a pole strength program will not result in increased strength or power. This goes back to the principle of adaptation. In order for the body to respond with an increase in strength gains, it must first be stressed beyond its current level of homeostasis. Sets of exercises

Table 5.3: Training Methodology for Pole	
What to Do	What to Avoid
• Train on the pole • Use weight training as a tool for physiological balance • Low to moderate aerobic activity for enjoyment and variation • Use intense sets of 10-15 repetitions to improve anaerobic endurance	• Consistent aerobic training • Excessive training in formats apart from pole • Designated strength programs with sets containing more than 12 repetitions

that include more than 15 repetitions before the athlete fatigues do not induce strength increases because the level of resistance does not place enough stress on the body to warrant strength adaptation. Exercise sets with 10-15 repetitions before fatigue can induce anaerobic endurance if intensity is high enough, which would be helpful for pole, but sets of 20+ repetitions (i.e. 30 crunches) induce aerobic endurance adaptations which can be counterproductive to a pole training program (4).

- **Frequency**

There are numerous cultural imperatives that suggest that the more an athlete trains, the bigger and faster their performance gains will be. Sayings such as "push through the pain" and "rest is for the weak" imply that doing more is the best way to get positive results. Unfortunately, these popular training messages are fundamentally flawed and can lead to destructive symptoms of overtraining and burnout. To determine how much a person should train we must once again go back to the principles of adaptation and supercompensation. As mentioned earlier, supercompensation is just a way to describe the different stages of the process of physiological adaptation. This is best described with the supercompensation curve on the following page.

An athlete's position on this curve will dictate when and how often they train. As seen on the curve, Phase III of supercompensation is the time when an increased level of homeostasis has been reached after fatigue is experienced from applied training stress (Phase I) and compensation through recovery occurs (Phase II). Although the time required to reach a level of increased performance is determined by several factors, Phase III of the supercompensation curve generally occurs 36 to 72 hours after an average training stimulus is applied. This phase is marked by a withdrawal of muscle soreness, a return of energy and strength, and

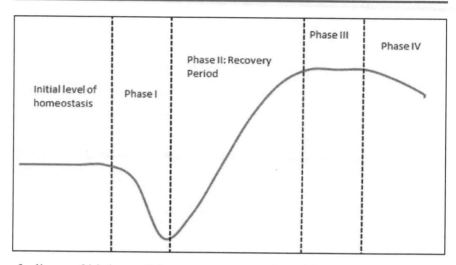

feelings of high confidence, energy, and positive thinking. This is the optimal time to apply another training stimulus as the body is now prepared to experience additional stress without becoming overloaded. In practical terms this means that a major muscle group should only be significantly trained every two to three days. For a pole athlete training in intermediate to advanced technique, two to three moderately intense, 1-2 hour sessions per week would be optimum for performance enhancement. A very important point to remember here is that this frequency and the associated time it takes for the body to reach Phase III of the supercompensation curve are hugely dependent on the volume and intensity of the training stimulus. The longer and harder an athlete trains during a session, the longer it will take for the body to recover and compensate. A pole athlete who trains particularly hard or long (as specified by their own physiological abilities and athletic level) will need to decrease the amount of times they train each week. To determine exactly how often to train, body and performance awareness can be used to gauge where the athlete is on the supercompensation curve. As a reminder, it is also important that the training sessions from week to week are varied and that additional time is taken off from training periodically to avoid overtraining.

- **Warm-up, Cool-down, and Stretching**

As tempting as it is to spend an entire pole training session working on tricks or technique, an adequate warm-up and cool-down are necessary and beneficial components of a productive workout. A warm-up benefits the athlete by literally elevating muscle temperature. It is believed that this, along with an increase in the amount of oxygen delivered to muscles, increases nerve conduction rate and metabolic reactions. This leads to higher power output due to faster, more forceful muscle contraction (4). Warm muscles and a training focused mindset generated during a warm-up can also help prevent injury during a training session. A warm-up should consist of a portion of low intensity general activity followed by slightly increased intensity activity that is specific to the type of training planned. For example, a pole warm-up may consist of 10-15 minutes of light calisthenics, floor work, and/or dynamic stretching followed by basic pole spins, climbing, or choreography with the pole. The warm-up should not, however, include static stretching (2,4,28). This type of stretching is most beneficial when muscles are warm and at least slightly fatigued. When this is the case, muscle spindles are less responsive to stretch, allowing the muscle to be stretched, cooled, and relaxed more thoroughly. In a "cold" muscle, the stretch reflex is heightened and the potential for pulling or tearing a muscle during static stretching is much greater. Dynamic stretches, such as shoulder circles, are a good option during the warm-up as they serve to warm the joints and muscle through movement.

The best time to practice static stretching is during the cool-down after the main portion of the training session. A cool-down allows the body to smoothly transition from a state of stress to rest and should consist of a portion of low intensity activity followed by static stretching. Static stretching at this time can be very beneficial to an athlete's training program as it can significantly improve flexibility and range of motion, decrease delayed onset muscle soreness, and increase rate of recovery (1,2,4). An adequate cool-down after a pole training session may consist of 5-10 minutes of lite calisthenics, dance, or floor work followed by 10-20 minutes of static stretching.

Putting it all Together

Between goals, training cycles, phases, multilateral development, intensity, volume, frequency, metabolic systems, stress/recovery relationships, intuition, body awareness, psychological and psychosocial influence, training methodology, and warm-ups and cool-downs, it can be easy to get lost in the weeds and overwhelmed when trying to create an individualized training plan. This is one of the reasons why so many people tend to flock to pre-designed generic programs or rely on popular fitness fads and cultural imperatives to direct their training. Don't let the variables in a training program scare you. It's true. All of the information and variables that go into designing an optimal program can be tremendous and complicated, but the ultimate goal is to simplify training design by accounting for all of these elements through body awareness and intuition. This results in a scientifically sound, individualized training program that doesn't require copious amounts of time designing or maintaining.

On the following pages are a few examples of typical training weeks with different overall focuses. These and the recommendations in the previous sections can help guide you in creating an individualized program while you become more sensitive to your own body's process of stress recovery and adaptation. Remember that these are only examples meant to help summarize the pole training suggestions made. These should not be treated as exercise prescriptions as each individual athlete is unique in their training and recovery needs. As you become more in tune with your body, you will be able to practice a more and more personalized, loose training program. Emphasis will shift from specifically directed phases and volumes of training to a more intuitive approach. The specific training suggestions and principles mentioned above are important concepts for an athlete, but they only attempt to direct athletic training by mimicking the intuition and guidance that the body gives. If these intuitions can't yet be accessed, use periodized training and the training logs on the following pages to guide you while you learn how to rely on your body for training direction. If you practice awareness throughout your training program, you will begin to recognize body signals congruent with the principles of adaptation and periodization. Eventually these signals can be relied on to guide training in the place of a prescribed schedule or program.

Phase of Annual Plan: Preparatory							
	Sunday	Monday	Tuesday	Wednesday	Thursday	Friday	Saturday
Training Routine		Calisthenics Floor work Dance/choreography stretching		Climbing Pole sits and laybacks Basic inversions Focus on technique		Hatha Yoga	Strength exercises for balance (reverse flys, lat pulls, wrist ext, flexion, assisted pole pull-ups, squats)
Energy level Motivation Psychological stress level Fatigue	Feeling a bit sluggish... glad to rest for the day	Feeling good and energized...was nice to move my body!	Little tired	Motivated for pole!		Was a bit stressed after work...rest and yoga helped	Energized before workout and ready to move
Soreness Bruising Niggles Sharp pains Presence of persistent injury			Little bit sore from calisthenics yesterday but doesn't feel like injury	Poling felt good...legs are a little bruised	Still a bit sore and bruised	Feeling much better and bruises are fading	Felt good. Will probably be sore tomorrow.
Overall performance		Had fun dancing... came up with some new choreography		Did really well! Practiced keeping legs straight inverting			Worked out until I felt pretty tired

Phase of **Annual Plan:** Competitive Phase

	Sunday	Monday	Tuesday	Wednesday	Thursday	Friday	Saturday
Training Routine	Advanced pole tricks focusing on technique Work on perfecting tricks			Practice competition routine – build endurance Focus on fluidity		Hatha Yoga	Practice new tricks and spins Strength balance exercises
Energy level Motivation Psychological stress level Feelings of fatigue	Felt good but worn out after pole	Tired from yesterday but excited about my progress	Energy and excitement growing... excited to pole tomorrow		Felt good to rest. I was a bit drained after practice yesterday	Stressed after a long day at work!	Don't have as much energy and motivation as I would like
Soreness Bruising Niggles or Twinges Sharp pains Presence of persistent injury	Some random bruising	Little bit sore		Feeling good!	Some soreness in my biceps, triceps, and mid back. Legs are bruised	Still a little sore. Yoga felt good.	Slight twinge of pain during full bracket hold. Will rest for a couple days
Overall performance	Got a couple advanced tricks down on my left side for the first time			Was able to get through the whole routine once. Need to work on fluidity			Performed well but stopped early I felt a small sharp pain in by forearm

		Sunday	Monday	Tuesday	Wednesday	Thursday	Friday	Saturday
Phase of Annual Plan: Transition								
Training Routine			Nia – expressive dance		Light weight training Stretching			Mixed level Pole Class
Energy level Motivation Psychological stress level Feelings of fatigue		Felt nice to lay around all day...was feeling worn out!	Medium energy level... body was feeling stiff before Nia	Starting to feel more rested	Feeling energized! Ready for some resistance training		Excited about pole class tomorrow. Came up with some new choreography to try	Had a blast in class!
Soreness Bruising Niggles or Twinges Sharp pains Presence of persistent injury				Got a blister on my foot from dancing yesterday				
Overall performance			Took it easy during class...felt good to wiggle and move		No problems			Learned some new choreography and practiced some old

	Sunday	Monday	Tuesday	Wednesday	Thursday	Friday	Saturday
Training Routine							
Energy level Motivation Psychological stress level Feelings of fatigue							
Soreness Bruising Niggles or Twinges Sharp pains Presence of persistent injury							
Overall performance							

Continuing Education Questions

1. Why is it important to have training or performance goals?
2. What does periodization provide for an athletic training program?
3. What are the three phases of an annual monocycle and what is the focus of each of these?
4. Why is intuition and body awareness important in training?
5. At what level do training practices begin to require more careful consideration and implementation?
6. What is the first step in any training program?
7. How often should a pole athlete train? What factors go into making this decision?
8. When is the best time to practice static stretching?
9. How can an athlete use intuition and body awareness to guide their athletic training program?

References and Additional Sources

1. Allerheiligeni, W. B. (1994). Stretching and warm-up. In T. R. Baechle (Ed.), Essentials of strength training and conditioning (pp. 289-313). Champaign, IL: Human Kinetics.
2. Blakey, W. P. (1994). Stretching without pain. Sechelt, B.C.: Twin Eagles Educational & Healing Institute.
3. Bompa, T. O., & Cornacchia, L. (2003). Serious strength training (2nd ed., pp. 3-66). Champaign, IL: Human Kinetics.
4. Bompa, T. O., & Haff, C. G. (2009). Periodization: Theory and methodology of training (5th ed.). Champaign, IL: Human Kinetics.
5. Bryant, C. X., & Green, D. J. (2010). ACE's essentials of exercise science for fitness professionals. San Diego, CA: American Council on Exercise.
6. DeAndrade, J. R., Grant, C., & Dixon, A. S. (1965). Joint distention and reflex muscle inhibition in the knee. Journal of

Bone and Joint Surgery, (47), 313-322.

7. Dudley, G. A., & Djamil, R. (1985). Incompatibility of endurance and strength training modes of exercise. Journal of Applied Physiology, (59), 255-269.

8. Foss, M. L., & Keteyian, S. J. (1998). Fox's physiological basis for exercise and sport. (6th ed., pp. 106-158). Boston, MA: WCB/McGraw-Hill.

9. Fry, A. C. (1998). The role of training intensity in resistance exercise overtraining and overreaching. In R. B. Kreider, A. C. Fry, & M. L. O'Toole (Eds.), Overtraining in sport (pp. 116-117). Champaign, IL: Human Kinetics.

10. Fry, A. C., Barnes, J. M., Kraemer, W. J., & Lynch, J. M. (1996). Overuse Syndrome of The Knees With High Intensity Resistance Exercise Overtraining: A Case Study 762. Medicine & Science in Sports & Exercise, 28(Supplement), 128. doi: 10.1097/00005768-199605001-00760

11. Hatfield, B. D., & Brody, E. B. (1994). The psychology of athletic preparation and performance: The mental management o physical resources. In T. R. Baechle (Ed.), Essentials of strength training and conditioning (pp. 163-185). Champaign, IL: Human Kinetics.

12. Hickson, R. C. (1980). Interference of strength development by simultaneously training for strength and endurance. European Journal of Applied Sport Science Research, (45), 255-269.

13. Holloway, J. B. (1994). Individual differences and their implications for resistance training. In T. R. Baechle (Ed.), Essentials of strength training and conditioning (pp. 151-161). Champaign, IL: Human Kinetics.

14. Kraemer, W. J., & Nindl, B. C. (1998). Factors involved with overtraining for strength and power. In R. B. Kreider, A. C. Fry, & M. L. O'Toole (Eds.), Overtraining in sport (pp. 69-86). Champaign, IL: Human Kinetics.

15. Kreider, R. B. (1998). Central fatigue hypothesis and over-training. In R. B. Kreider, A. C. Fry, & M. L. O'Toole (Eds.), Overtraining in sport (pp. 309-331). Champaign, IL: Human Kinetics.

16. Kreider, R. B., Fry, A. C., & O'Toole, M. L. (1998). Over-training in sport. Champaign, IL: Human Kinetics.

17. Kreider, R. B., Miriel, V., & Bertun, E. (1993). Amino acid supplementation and exercise performance. Sports Medicine, 16(3), 190-209. doi: 10.2165/00007256-199316030-00004

18. Meyers, A. W., & Whelan, J. P. (1998). A systemic model for understanding psychosocial influences in overtraining. In R. B. Kreider, A. C. Fry, & M. L. O'Toole (Eds.), Overtraining in sport (pp. 335-369). Champaign, IL: Human Kinetics.

19. Newsholme, E. A., Parry-Billings, M., McAndrew, M., & Budgett, R. (1991). Biochemical mechanism to explain some characteristics of overtraining (F. Brouns, Ed.). Medical Sports Science Advances in Nutrition and Top Sport, 32, 79-93.

20. Parry-Billings, M., Blomstrand, E., McAndrew, N., & News-holme, E. (1990). A communicational link between skeletal muscle, brain, and cells of the immune system. International Journal of Sports Medicine, 11(S 2), S122-S128. doi: 10.1055/s-2007-1024863

21. Rountree, S. H. (2011). The athlete's guide to recovery: Rest, relax, and restore for peak performance. Boulder, CO: Ve-loPress.

22. Sherman, K. S., Shakespear, D. T., Stokes, M., & Young, A. (1983). Inhibition of voluntary quadriceps activity after meni-sectomy. Clinical Science, (64), 70.

23. Stone, M. H., Stone, M., & Sands, B. (2007). Principles and practice of resistance training. Champaign, IL: Human Kinet-ics.

24. Wathen, D. (1994). Muscle balance. In T. R. Baechle (Ed.),

Essentials of strength training and conditioning (pp. 424-429). Champaign, IL: Human Kinetics.

25. Wathen, D. (1994). Periodization: Concepts and applications. In T. R. Baechle (Ed.), Essentials of strength training and conditioning (pp. 459-472). Champaign, IL: Human Kinetics.

26. Wathen, D. (1994). Training frequency. In T. R. Baechle (Ed.), Essentials of strength training and conditioning (pp. 455-458). Champaign, IL: Human Kinetics.

27. Wathen, D. (1994). Training volume. In T. R. Baechle (Ed.), Essentials of strength training and conditioning (pp. 447-450). Champaign, IL: Human Kinetics.

28. Woods, K., Bishop, P., & Jones, E. (2007). Warm-up and stretching in the prevention of muscular injury. Sports Medicine, 37(12), 1089-1099. doi: 10.2165/00007256-200737120-00006

Conclusion

Today is an exciting time for vertical sport and dance. As more people are exposed to pole, its many physical, psychological, and social benefits are experienced and shared. As part of a new and quickly growing sport, members of the pole community are in a fantastic position to influence and mold perspectives on and application of training methodology. As pole athletes, we have the opportunity to dismiss typical negative and harmful exercise practices and cultural imperatives by gaining and applying knowledge of sports physiology, principles of training and adaptation, overtraining, program design, and the application of body awareness. By capitalizing on this opportunity, we will not only optimize our own individual training and performance but will also reinforce and sustain the positive, encouraging, and enjoyable environment that so many love about pole.

Learning and applying the many factors that make up a good training program can seem scary and overwhelming, but at its foundation, productive training is simple. During recovery, the body adapts to stress previously applied to it. If recovery time is sufficient, performance gains will occur. If another training stimulus is consistently applied before recovery is complete, decreases in performance and other overtraining symptoms will develop. Specific training program design can be further guided by the performance goals of the athlete, bioenergetics, and periodization concepts. The most important thing to remember about training is that our bodies are designed with an acute awareness of the conditions that they are experiencing. The human body is intricately wired to know precisely when to go and when to stop. If we listen, our bodies will tell us exactly where they are in the cycle of supercompensation. The whole industry of legitimate athletic training is focused on identifying and describing these moments because the most superior athletic development occurs when training is timed precisely with the readiness of the body. Researchers and coaches spend enormous amounts of time and money to find out exactly when and how much a person should train. The reason they have such difficulty is because each person is different. People recover at different rates, they have different physiological make ups, they experience varying levels of stress throughout their daily lives, and they have different training and exercise histories. When it comes down to it, only the individual has the ability to know and experience exactly where they are at in the stress/adaptation continuum. If a person can put away all of the unscientific cultural training demands and access this knowledge through an intimate relationship with their own body and the messages it sends, then they are in a most superior position to become an amazing vertical athlete.

About the Author

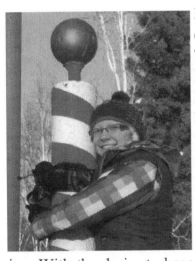

Bethany Freel is an American Council on Exercise certified Personal Trainer, PoleMoves certified Pole Instructor, and Nia (Neuromuscular Integrative Action) white belt. She has lived in Alaska for the last 11 years where she is an engineer and pole instructor. Bethany has been involved in athletics and strength training for much of her life from recreational and competitive sport to compulsive training and overtraining. With the desire to become a superb, fit athlete, she worked out long and hard. She always ran the extra mile and pushed through the pain, only to see stagnated results and persistent injury. Through research, experiences in pole and training, and a journey of personal growth, she has emerged from the damaging and unnecessary practice of overtraining with a passion for learning and spreading the word regarding optimum training practice, overtraining, intuitive-ness in exercise, and body respect.

Made in the USA
San Bernardino, CA
04 June 2015